Tony Funge's

Great Temptations

over 150 delicious, tasty recipes using the More, or Less dietary guidelines

Marlin Publications
Wheelers Hill, Victoria

Life. Be in it.

First published in 1989 by
Marlin Publications
741 Ferntree Gully Road Wheelers Hill Victoria 3150 Australia
and 18 Anne Street Smithfield Heights North Queensland 4878 Australia

Funge, Tony, 1945– .
Tony Funge's great temptations.

Includes index.
ISBN 1 875165 02 9.

1. Reducing diets — Recipes. 2. Salt-free diet — Recipes. 3. Low-cholesterol diet — Recipes. 4. Sugar-free diet — Recipes. I. Title. II. Title: Great temptations : over 150 delicious tasty recipes . . .

641.5′63

Photography Phyl Wymant
Designed by Peter Yates
Edited by Janet M Henderson
Typeset by Abb-typesetting Pty Ltd, Collingwood, Victoria
Printed by Brown Prior Anderson, Burwood, Victoria

Contents

Dedication

This book is dedicated to my fantastic partner, friend, and wife, Joan Maree Funge. Joan has been the driving force and ideas person behind all my ventures and a tremendous help with this book.

Foreword

Everybody has heard of '**Life. Be in it**', and our popular message has been broadcast all over Australia, and indeed, overseas too.

Our main aim — for the past 15 years — has been to promote a fitter, healthier and happier Australia. Now, '**Life. Be in it**' in association with Marlin Publications, is delighted to present the '**Life. Be in it**' **Cookbook**.

This cookbook is the product of many hours of hard work by renowned chef, Tony Funge, and he has based the recipes on the highly successful More, or Less Diet. The diet promotes the idea that you should eat *more* of the high fibre, nutritious foods and *less* of the sugary, salty foods. Tony has used this philosophy in creating these recipes, and clearly, it *is* possible to create 'Great Temptations' that are enticing, tasty, and — most important — good for your diet!

The cookbook contains over 150 exciting recipes which, I feel sure, you will love making; and rest assured, they *will* benefit your health!

We *must* learn to eat healthier and more nutritious foods.

I hope that one day, Norm, the '**Life. Be in it**' anti-hero, will try some of these recipes.

I commend to you the '**Life. Be in it**' **Cookbook**!
Happy eating.

Yours in Life,

DR IAN BENNETT
Chief Executive

Life. Be in it.

Preface

What you eat has a great effect on your health. The More, or Less Diet encourages you to eat *more* foods which are beneficial to good health and *less* of those which are low in nutrition.

This means more bread, cereals, vegetables and fruit, and less foods with fat, salt, added sugar and less alcohol. By following this plan, not only will you feel better, but you will lessen your chance of being affected by disease which can be linked to your diet.

These disorders include heart disease, stroke, some cancers, diabetes, liver and gall bladder problems, and dental caries.

Acknowledgements

There are so many people who have assisted me, in one way or another with this book; accordingly it gives me much pleasure to thank them. Dr Ian Bennett, Dr Jack Cygler, Dr Meridith Taylor, Ken Adcock, Ross Woodward and the wonderful people at '**Life. Be in it**', whose weight management team graciously provided the information section concerning weight management, and gave me so much time, assistance and encouragement.

Peter Yates for his design work, and Janet Henderson who edited the manuscript. The Commonwealth Department of Health; Phyl Wymant for his brilliant photography; Gordon Porter and Gwen Bowditch for their assistance with the photographic sessions. Kerrin O'Connor, of Image Interiors, Mornington, who generously supplied the accessories for those photographic sessions.

Debbie Williams for her typing; somehow she managed to understand my writing and scribble.

To Panasonic, for allowing the use of their marvellous juice extractor; and a very special thank you to Suzanne Porter, whose persistence and dedication in putting this whole package together was nothing short of remarkable.

Introduction

My career as a chef was a foregone conclusion; almost from the time I was born. At the age of 15, I began my apprenticeship at the Ritz Restaurant, Lonsdale Street, Melbourne, where I undertook 5 years of training to become a qualified chef. This was coupled with one day per week, at the William Angliss College. Although the days and nights were long, I loved the work so much that the Ritz decided to send me to Europe for additional experience.

I joined the staff at the Hotel Quirinale in Rome, which fine-tuned my Ritz training. On my return to Melbourne, I gained as much experience as possible over the next few years, achieving several awards: Apprentice of the Year and the coveted William Angliss College Bronze Medallion. The College then approached me to teach the up-and-coming chefs of Australia and pass my expertise on to them.

After preparing conventional recipes in my restaurants, 'The Treble Clef', Melbourne; 'Sharkey's', Noosa; 'Scampi's, Mornington and 'The Bay Cottage', Frankston; by 1983, Joan and I had in fact changed our diet to a healthier one and seriously considered opening a restaurant with the concept of no fat, salt or sugar.

We opened 'Eat Naturally' in Frankston in 1983 and adapted many of our conventional recipes to fit in with these dietary guidelines. It was a brilliant success. We were amazed at the number of patrons who would travel many kilometres to eat with us and purchase meals to freeze at home and eat later. We thought we were the only people who had changed our way of eating.

By 1985 we opened 'Fungies' Restaurant in Toorak. The demand was phenomenal. 'Fungies' served over 3000 patrons per week, 7 days and nights.

It made me realise just how important it is to have the right recipe selections and to follow a healthy eating plan. I have taken the highly successful '**Life. Be in it**' More, or Less Diet and modified my recipes for this book, to share my favourites with you. We hope they will be enjoyed by all who use them. Good health is no luxury, but a natural part of life.

Bon Appétit
Tony Funge

Life. Be in it.™

Weight management

The purpose of this chapter is to provide a brief overview to the issue of weight management in the Australian population and to examine the ways in which the problem can be addressed.

Everyone reaches a time in life when they realise they are not immortal, and to remain in good health and have a long life will require some change in diet and lifestyle. Each of us has the ultimate responsibility to determine our own health and well being. Whether we chose to look after ourselves or continue to engage in behaviour that may eventually be detrimental to health, is our choice, and we must accept the consequences. Good eating patterns should be established from birth, so until children become responsible for their own health, parents must assume the responsibility for the eating and exercise habits of their young.

In our society, food is freely available and often consumed inappropriately. We eat for many reasons; habit, social pressure, cultural expectations, personal preference and, because we are so busy, convenience. Combine these factors with a sedentary existence, and we have a significant proportion of the population with weight problems, suffering the health consequences of being overweight or obese.

The concept of weight management entails examining your lifestyle, including your dietary habits and activity levels. It involves making a personal commitment to improve that lifestyle in the long term. It requires a balanced positive attitude; short-term obsessions with strict dieting, are never sustained. After all, food is a pleasurable part of life, and eating an enjoyable pastime. What we should strive for is a balance where we enjoy the 'right' foods, *most* of the time and the high kilojoule (high fat, high sugar), foods *less* of the time.

The same balance needs to be struck for our levels of activity. It is *not* necessary to attend aerobics classes seven times a week to achieve a good level of cardiovascular fitness. Three or 4 quick walks a week for 30 minutes are adequate.

So let us examine the overweight effects on the individual and society, and *then* look at constructive ways of remedying the situation.

The problems of being overweight and why they occur

The statistics relating to the proportion of overweight and obese individuals in Australia are disturbing. Overall, 43 per cent of men and 35 per cent of women are either overweight or obese. Further studies have revealed that 50 per cent of men aged 35 and over, and 50 per cent of women aged 50 and over, are overweight.

The consequences of being overweight are naturally of concern to those affected, but there are also implications for society at large.

For the overweight person, the consequences can be broadly classified into *Physical* and *Nonphysical* effects.

Physical: there are a number of diseases which are either caused by or exacerbated by excess weight. These include heart disease, hypertension, strokes, diabetes, liver and gall bladder disorders, degenerative joint disease (arthritis, gout), back problems, some cancers, hernias, varicose veins, sleep apnoea, or surgical complications. Of course there are phsycial discomforts, such as shortness of breath, decreased mobility and indigestion. Studies have also shown that overweight or obese individuals have a higher rate of accidents.

Nonphysical: many emotional problems are associated with being overweight. In an 'image conscious' society, fat people often suffer decreased self esteem, lack of confidence, difficulty obtaining jobs, insecurity in social settings and difficulty buying clothes. They also pay higher life insurance premiums.

The impact on society as a whole is due to increased health-care costs for the conditions associated with being overweight: costs related to payment of sickness and invalidity benefits, and reduced earnings.

What is fat and how do we become overweight?
Fat is stored energy. When we eat too much and exercise too little, the surplus energy is converted into fat. However, fat does perform useful functions within the body:

- it insulates us against the cold
- it protects organs within our body
- it acts as an energy reserve if we are without food e.g., illness and famine
- it makes hormones e.g., oestrogen

Fat is stored in fat cells called adipocytes. Our body fat increases when either:

- the fat cells grow in size, *or*
- the number of fat cells increase

Much is still unknown about how fat cells develop. Many fat cells are formed *in utero* during the third trimester of pregnancy. This process continues during the first few years of life and during pre-adolescence.

Fat children become fat adults when too much fat is gained during the early years. Thus, a fat child will have many more fat cells than a lean child. These extra fat cells remain for life, which means the fat child will more likely have a battle with body fat as an adult.

Weight gain out of these critical periods of fat cell development generally results in an increase in the *size* of the fat cell, not the number of cells.

However, in extreme cases of obesity developing in adults, an increase in cells may also occur because the overloaded existing cells are unable to store any further fat.

Genetics is a factor in determining whether we are fat. The number of fat cells we have is, to a degree, inherited. However, we seem only to inherit the tendency to be overweight. Whether we do or not is more dependent on environmental factors.

When we study the distribution of fat on the body, it is evident that there are two main body types: Gynoid and Android.

Gynoid: this is the 'pear shape' as fat tends to accumulate in the hips, buttocks, thighs and lower abdomen. Women may have this body type.

Android: fat is located on the back, shoulders and upper abdomen. This body shape has an increased risk of cardiovascular problems, and is associated with higher blood cholesterol and lipid levels; also diabetes, high blood pressure and gout. The good news is that it responds readily to diet and exercise.

Your body type *is* your body type. It is not possible to predict which part of your body will lose fat. Women lose weight generally more easily from the trunk, but the thighs tend to be more resistant. Of course, with fat loss, the general line of the body will improve and the exaggeration will be less marked. Exercise improves muscle tone, but it is not possible to lose fat in one particular area and spare the rest of the body.

A classic example of the myth of the 'spot fat' reduction is the hype surrounding cellulite. Cellulite is stored fat in fat cells i.e., it is just another term for fat! Cellulite reduction will occur when combining sensible dieting with exercise but there are NO genuine nonsurgical methods of removing fat cells, despite claims to the contrary.

How much fat is too much? i.e., how to determine an acceptable weight

How do you determine whether or not you have a weight problem? The most common method used to gauge an acceptable weight is a height and weight chart.

Height-for-weight tables are usually derived from insurance company statistics; hence they reflect the best weight for a long life and good health.

If your weight falls within the recommended range, then it is acceptable, and generally could not be considered a health problem. A possible exception is an individual at the upper limit of the recommended range with medical problems such as hypertension, back problems, diabetes or high lipid levels. He/she might well benefit from further weight loss.

Note that on these charts there is no reference to age. It is neither acceptable nor sensible for our weight to increase with age. We should endeavour to maintain the same 'ideal' weight for life.

There is also a formula which relates a person's height to weight and provides an indication of the degree of that weight problem. This formula is the Body Mass Index (BMI). You can calculate your own BMI by dividing your weight in kilograms by the square of your height in metres i.e., $BMI = Wt\ kg/(Ht\ m)^2$. Compare your BMI with the following table:

DESCRIPTIVE TERM	MEN	WOMEN
Underweight	Less than 19	Less than 18
Acceptable Weight	20–25	19–24
Overweight	26–30	25–30
Obese	Over 30	Over 30

The BMI is an accurate guide for most of the population. As with height-for-weight charts there are exceptions: those with excess muscle bulk (weight lifters, heavy manual labourers etc.), who are heavy but not necessarily overweight. Therefore the BMI should only be considered in the context of a person's general level of activity.

A more precise way of determining how overweight you are is to measure how much body fat you have. This is done by having a 4-site 'pinch-test' using an instrument called a skin calliper.

Body measurements

There are even more sophisticated ways of measuring body fat such as determining the body density (weight compared with volume), and by measuring body weight underwater and the amount of water it displaces in a tank. Ultrasonic techniques may be used to determine body fat as well as the injection of water-soluble substances (which only penetrate lean tissues, not fat issues), and subsequent measurement of the level of the substance in the blood stream.

Least sophisticated, but perhaps most revealing, is a test you can perform at home. Remove your clothes, stand in front of a full length mirror and take a good look at yourself . . .

Diet

SORTING THROUGH THE CONFUSION

With hundreds of diets, diet books and articles on weight loss it is very confusing for the average person to decide which diet to use in order to lose weight.

Every time a new diet appears — everyone seems to try it. This exemplifies the attitude of many people to weight loss. You do *not* need a miracle new diet to achieve permanent weight loss! What you need is a sensible eating plan that suits your needs. Combine this with regular exercise and a change in eating habits and you will be able to achieve weight loss and maintain that loss.

Many fad and crash diets can, in fact, be dangerous. Be wary of those diets which claim to originate from reputable organisations and appear unbalanced or focus on particular foods to the exclusion of others. Similarly, there are no wonder potions or drugs that will magically melt fat away and allow you to eat whatever you want without putting on weight.

Experimenting with these unbalanced, very low calorie diets underlies many of the fears and misconceptions that overweight people have about the type of diet that is necessary to lose weight.

Examples of irrational fears are:

- diet food is bland and boring
- I will have to stick to a very strict diet in order to lose weight
- I will never be able to have high calorie foods or I will put on weight again.
- a diet must be a misery for it to be successful
- I will have to refuse all invitations or I will break my diet

Such fears are groundless. Worse still, they may be offered as excuses for not even attempting to lose weight.

Another source of confusion lies in what is a healthy diet and what is a weight reducing diet. A weight reducing diet should be healthy, but having a healthy diet may not necessarily enable you to lose weight — it depends on the balance of food consumed. In fact, many overwieght people do eat very well — low fat, low sugar, plenty of grains and cereals, fruit and vegetables etc. They may be eating just a little too much of the right foods and, over a long period, have gradually put on weight.

It is also important to be aware that certain foods promoted as healthier alternatives may be of little value in a weight reducing diet. Muesli bars may be as high in fat and sugars as a chocolate bar, and as kilojoule intense. Likewise, vegetable oils may not contain cholesterol but their kilojoule count is the same as butter. Nutritionally, honey and raw sugar are no different from white sugar and the kilojoule count is similar.

CHOOSING A HEALTHY WEIGHT REDUCING EATING PLAN

In choosing a healthy weight reducing eating plan, the two prime considerations are the types of foods eaten and the total number of kilojoules consumed.

The More, or Less Diet highlights in a simple way the sorts of foods we should be eating to achieve good health. We need to eat *more* of the foods high in nutrients — bread, cereals, and fruit, and *less* of foods low in nutrition — fats, sugar, alcohol and salt.

In considering the total number of kilojoules consumed, the majority of people will lose weight on 5000 kJ (1200 Kcal), per day. If you find that you do not lose on this amount try to increase your level of activity rather than cutting down on food intake. If your job is particularly physically active (e.g., manual labour) you may lose weight on 8400 kJ (2000 Kcal), a day. A safe and acceptable weight loss is ½–1 kg a week. This may not seem like much weight but it must be remembered that every 1 kg of fat represents approximately 30 000 kJ (7000 Kcal), of stored surplus energy.

The 5000 kJ should comprise a balance of foods from the 5 food groups in this book; fruit and vegetables, meat group, dairy group, bread and cereals, and fats. By selecting a balance of foods from these 5 groups you will receive all the energy nutrients that your body requires.

In summary, a balanced weight reduction diet might include the following selections from the food groups:

Breads and cereals (1000 kJ)	— 4 servings
one serving:	= ⅓ cup cooked rice *or* pasta
	= ½ cup cereal
	= 3 crispbreads
	= 1 slice wholemeal bread
Meat group (1200 kJ)	— 1½ servings
one serving:	= 75 g lean red meat
	= 90 g lean chicken *or* rabbit
	= 150 g fish
	= 2 eggs
	= ¾ cup cooked lentils, vegetable legumes
	= 30 g nuts
Dairy group (900 kJ)	— 3 servings
one serving:	= 200 ml skim milk
	= 200 g natural yoghurt, low fat
	= 20 g cheddar cheese
	=60 g cottage cheese, low fat
Fruit and vegetables	— 3 servings fruit (750 kJ)
	— 2 servings higher kJ vegetables (500 kJ)
one serving:	= 1 potato
	= ½ cup corn *or* peas
	— unlimited green and other vegetables
Fats (450 kJ)	— 3 servings
one serving:	= 1 level teaspoon butter, oil, margarine etc.

Having examined the components of a balanced eating plan, here are some important points to consider in tailoring that plan to suit your needs.

(a) Have the types of foods that you enjoy. Do not force yourself to eat

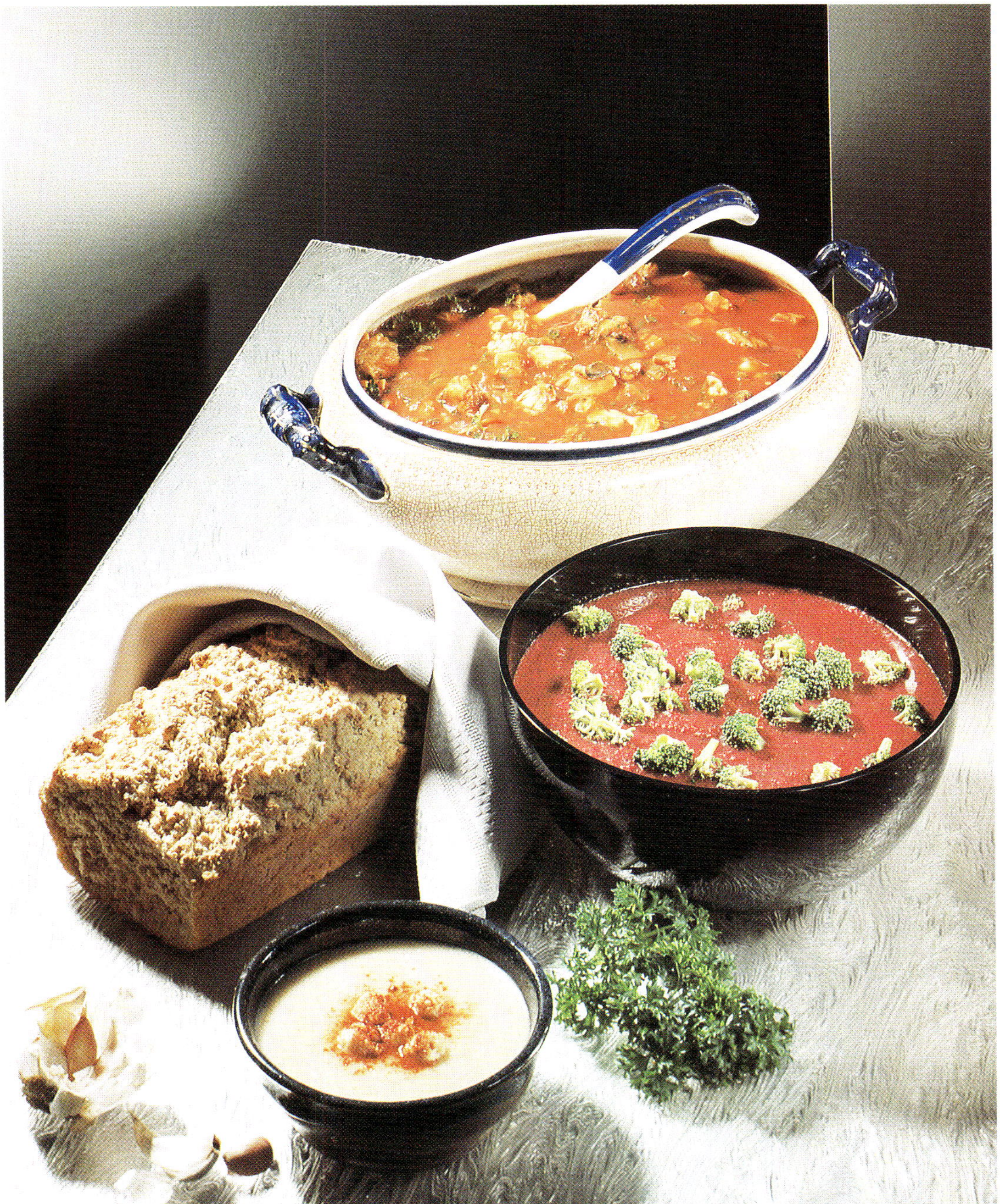

'Fishestrone' (*page 31*), Beetroot and broccoli broth (*page 26*)
'Cream' of cauliflower soup (*page 29*), Beer bread (*page 92*)

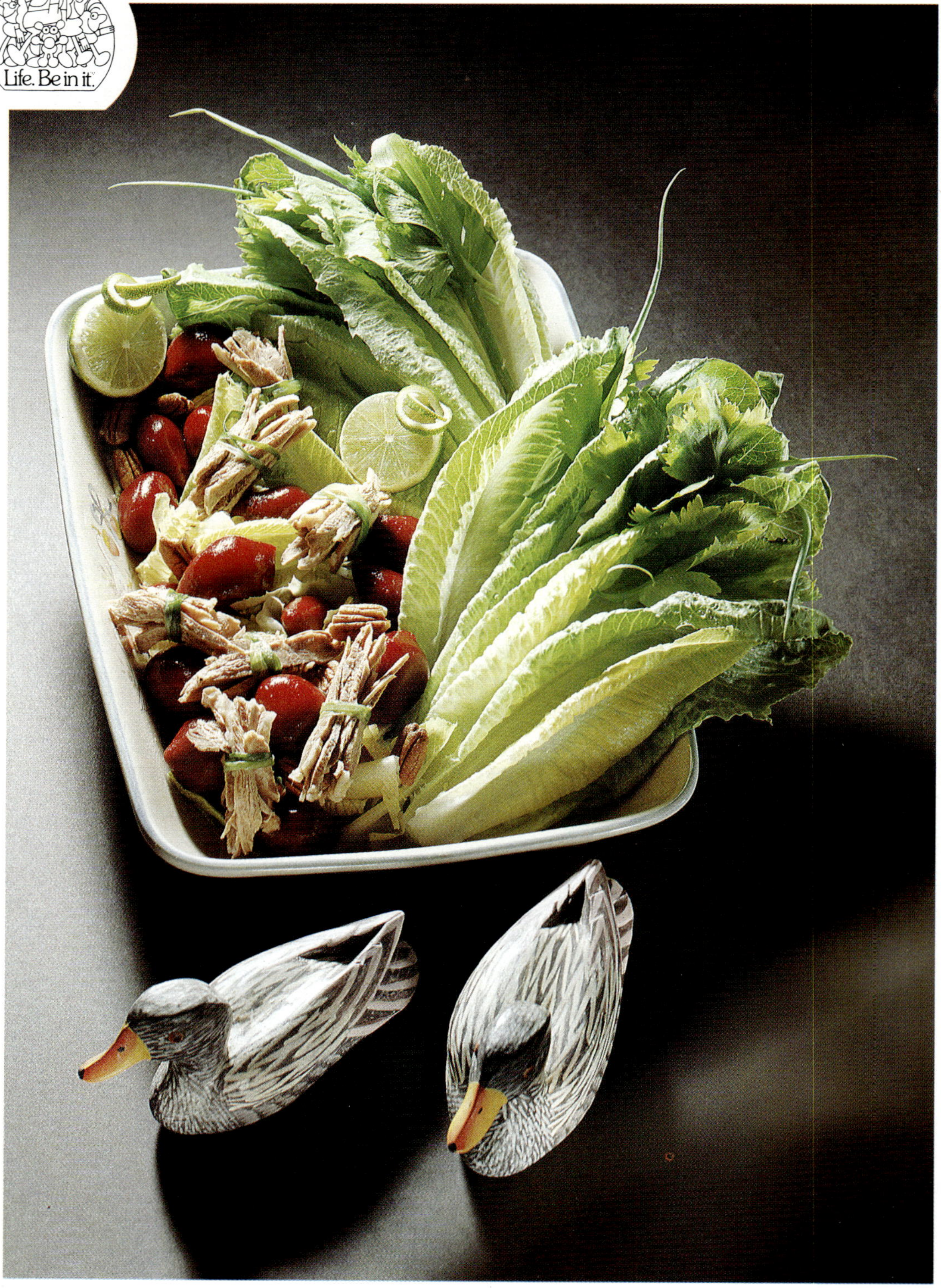

Duck salad with baby beetroot (*page 51*)

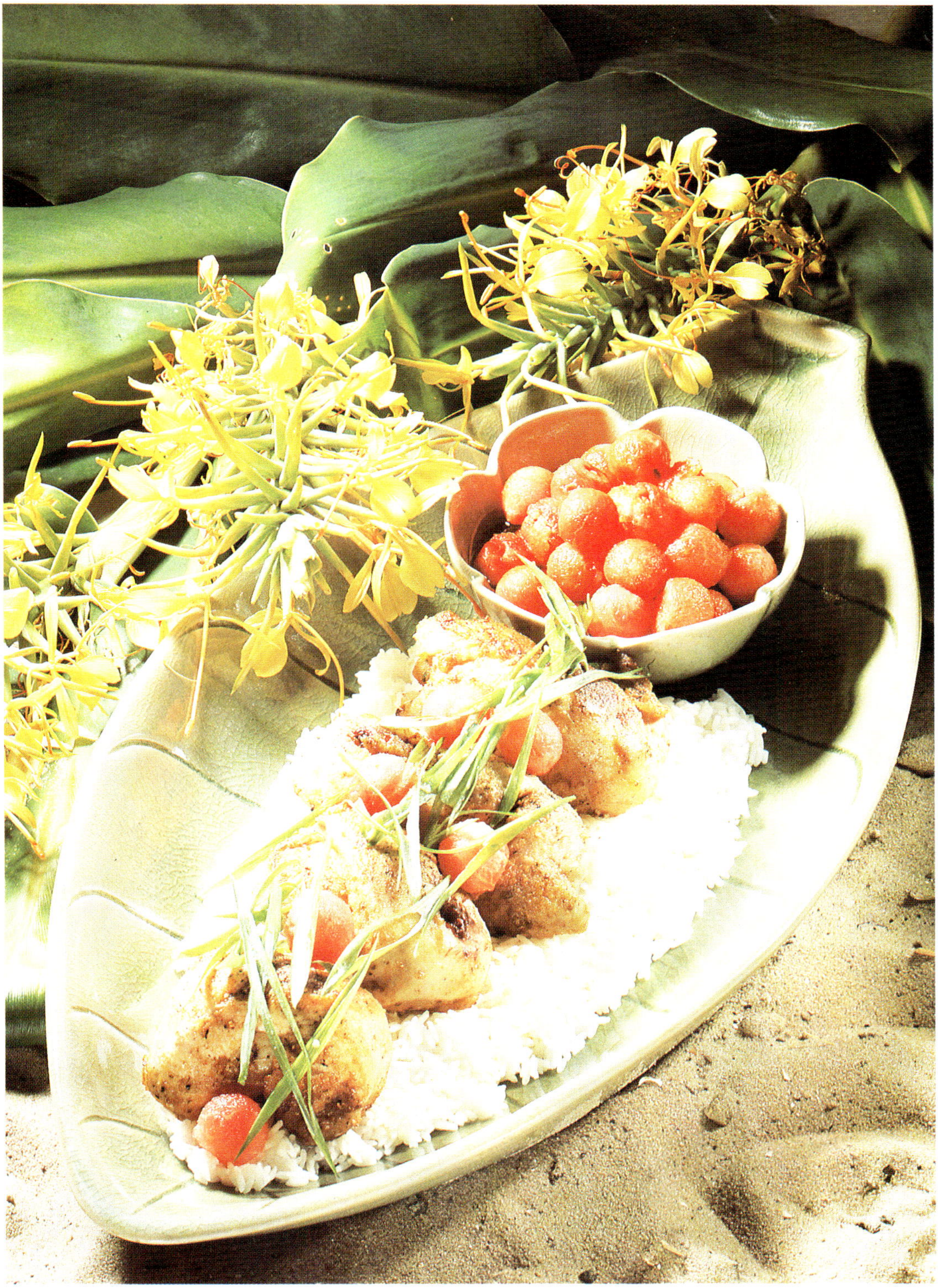

Ginger and tamari chicken (*page 52*)

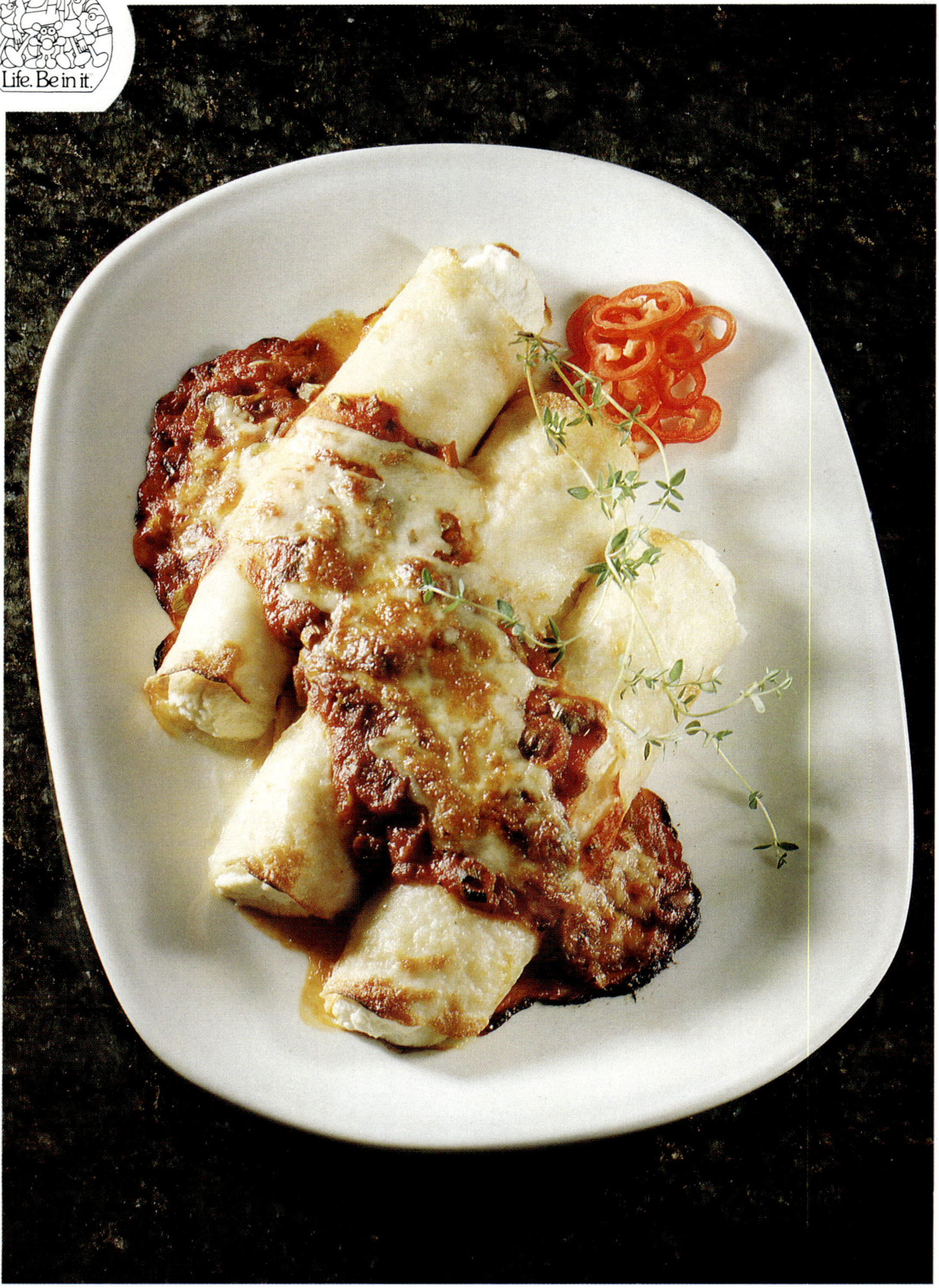

Vegetarian cannelloni (*page 120*)

foods you find unpalatable in the belief that they are healthy or low in kilojoules. Realistically, how long will you continue to follow an eating plan if you do not enjoy the foods?

(b) Devise your eating plan to suit yourself. Understand the combinations of foods that meet your particular energy needs and appetite. Be an active participant in designing your eating plan.

(c) Be adventurous and experiment with different foods and different means of cooking. As this cookbook wonderfully demonstrates, you need not rely on fats and sugars to give your food flavour.

(d) Use foods that are freely available and fit within your budget.

(e) Be organised. Plan the foods you wish to purchase and the meals that you will eat, in advance.

Spread your intake of foods over the day. Eat breakfast — the energy requirement of your body is greatest late morning and early afternoon. It makes sense, therefore, to have a solid breakfast and a good lunch. If you eat very little during the day and save all your food for the evening meal, your body will not use the food energy effectively. Ideally, the evening meal should be quite small.

Fruit or crispbreads make a perfect snack between meals. Bowls of vegetable soup are marvellous for reducing appetite and, if made from only vegetables, are very low in calories.

Water is an important element of a weight reducing diet. It reduces the appetite, helps to stimulate the excretion of waste products, improves the delivery of nutrients to the cells and reduces retention of fluids within the body. For people with normal kidneys, and no history of cardiac failure, at least 2 litres (8 glasses), should be consumed each day.

Do not consider yourself 'on a diet'. If you are 'on a diet' the implication is that one day you will be 'off the diet'. Think of yourself as following a life-long healthy eating plan. This life-long plan is flexible enough for you to enjoy high calorie foods in moderation, from time-to-time.

Finally, think positively about food by concentrating on all the good healthy foods you *may* eat instead of dwelling on the higher kilojoule foods you need to restrict for a while.

Exercise

Understandably, if you are overweight or obese you may have little inclination to exercise. Your body is already under the strain of carrying extra kilograms and you may feel lethargic from overeating.

However, an exercise regime will help your weight loss and in a number of ways improve your general state of well being.

There are two major areas where exercise will physically improve your body's ability to lose weight.

1 Regular exercise will alter the proportion of (lean) muscle-to-fat tissue in a positive direction. Fat tissue is sluggish and adversely affects the

metabolism of the body. Lean tissue uses up much more energy and thus increases the metabolism. If you undertake to diet without regular exercise, you will lose valuable lean (muscle) tissue as well as fat tissue. If you then regain the weight, only fat tissue is regained. Hence, even if you return to the same body weight as before the diet, more of the weight will be fat tissue because the metabolism is adversely affected by this greater amount of fat and the tendency is to become fatter. This is why repeated episodes of weight loss and weight gain, particularly without regular exercise, tends to make you fatter and fatter.

The positive effect that arises when exercise is combined with dieting is the increased amount of muscle tissue. Muscle tissue as we have said uses more energy, and hence, your metabolism functions at a higher level. This allows a bit more leeway with your diet and helps you to feel you are attacking the problem on two fronts.

2 When you exercise, metabolism is speeded up temporarily — for approximately 24 hours. Do not make the mistake of assuming that exercise will compensate for dietary indiscretion; it takes one hour of cycling to burn up a small piece of cheesecake! Hence, exercise without consciously watching your food intake will *not* achieve a successful weight loss.

Other beneficial effects of exercise include better regulation of appetite, looking and feeling fit and healthy, and cardiovascular fitness. Exercise is also an excellent means of stress management.

Having established that a regular exercise routine has many benefits on physical and emotional well being, let us examine the different types of exercise, and what level of exercise is desirable. The type of exercise you undertake should be appropriate to your degree of weight problem, age and general health. Without too much difficulty, this should fit agreeably into your lifestyle.

Any activity that involves movement of the body's large muscle groups is beneficial, and the more muscles involved the better.

Walking is an excellent form of exercise and is appropriate for most people. It should be performed briskly. It is particularly suitable for the very overweight; is cheap, gets you into the fresh air and away from the kitchen.

Other beneficial forms of exercise are bike riding (exercise or push bike), swimming, rowing, dancing, skipping, low-impact aerobics and water aerobics. Those who are very overweight should not jog or perform high-impact aerobics as these forms of exercise will cause great strain on joints and may result in injury. You should begin your program with short bursts, and gradually increase the time and intensity of your exercise. If you are over 35 or markedly overweight, consult your doctor for approval of the form of activity you have chosen. You *must* enjoy the form of exercise you have to undertake, otherwise how long will you continue to do it? Some people prefer to exercise with others in team sports; squash, aerobics classes etc. Others prefer to exercise alone.

If you work long hours it may be beneficial to have home exercise equipment e.g., an exercise bike or rowing machine that can easily fit into your lifestyle.

To gain aerobic benefit, you should try to exercise for 20–30 minutes, 3–4 times a week.

Do not make the mistake of thinking that because you are busy you are exercising efficiently. People such as nurses who are walking all day are not necessarily 'fit'. To get cardiovascular fitness and boost the metabolsim, the exercise needs to be sustained (and the pulse rate elevated), for 20–30 minutes — at least. However, any means you can find to increase your level of activity will be beneficial to you over a prolonged period. For instance, take the stairs instead of the lift; park the car at the furthest end of the car park; go for a short walk in your lunch break and walk to the local store instead of driving.

Behaviour modification

Much of the eating response is learned. Behavioural modification involves unlearning patterns of behaviour which many of us have adopted since childhood.

Any successful attempt to lose weight involves not only looking at the food we eat, but must also involve an examination of the many reasons why we eat.

Why do we eat? If people only ate when they were hungry — very few would be overweight. Overweight people eat as a response to a wide variety of cues. Studies have demonstrated that overweight individuals are more susceptible to external stimuli to eat than thin individuals. For instance, the overweight eat because they are stimulated by the availability of the sight and taste of food. This makes it difficult in a society such as ours where, for most people, food is freely available and promoted heavily on TV advertisements designed to send the late-night-snacker to the refrigerator or pantry.

Eating may also be stimulated by psychological factors. Food has a calming effect and may be sought as a response to pain, anxiety, arousal or excitement. Overweight people will eat as a response to these stimuli whereas thin people may lose their appetite entirely. Because the overweight often have low self esteem and may be insecure emotionally, this makes them even more sensitive to factors such as stress and anxiety.

If you are eating for comfort, try to recognise the underlying emotion or feeling that is compelling you to eat. Examples of such feelings are depression, loneliness, fear of rejection and anxiety. Once you have recognised what you are feeling, you will be able to be more objective, and there is less likelihood of reacting by eating. After all, eating may make you feel a little better in the short term, but ultimately, will not help you to solve any of your problems.

Develop alternative strategies to handle stress. For instance, exercise will increase your sense of well being and control. Learn the techniques of relaxation, meditation or deep breathing and use these if you are feeling anxious or overwhelmed. Confront problems directly that are troubling you. Practise being assertive and learn to say no without fear of rejection.

One of the commonest reasons given for eating is boredom. Being bored is not so much a problem of having nothing to do — after all most of us would have a long list of tasks we have been putting off addressing — but more a case of 'I can't be bothered'. Hence, we waste our valuable time by eating.

Occupy your free time by either fully relaxing or by tackling a task which would result in a productive and constructive utilisation of that time. It may be a task as simple as defrosting the refrigerator or washing the car, but once accomplished, there will be a sense of satisfaction in having achieved something worthwhile.

Now that you have become more discriminating about *why* you eat, also examine *how* you eat, where you eat your food, and the times of the day when your appetite is particularly difficult to control.

Do you eat too quickly? If you eat very quickly you will probably finish your meals not feeling pleasantly satisfied, but feeling bloated, uncomfortable and as though you have overeaten. It takes 20 minutes after you start eating for the appetite regulating centre in your brain to register that food has been eaten. Having soups as a starter at meals is an excellent way of allowing time for signals to reach your brain that food is being consumed. Slow down the rate at which you eat, put down your knife and fork between mouthfuls, chew thoroughly, and never use fingers for eating.

Always try to have your meals in one place and do no other activities at that place. For example, when eating at home, eat at the kitchen/dining table, not at your desk, at the refrigerator or on the sofa. Similarly, do not eat whilst you are engaged in other activities such as watching TV, reading a book, studying, or driving the car. When you are eating you need to be aware of it but if you are concentrating on another activity, you may not even know how much you are eating.

Be aware of any little eating rituals you may be engaging in, such as the doughnut and cappucino before work.

In summary, become aware of your eating behaviour, and when you have recognised your patterns of behaviour with foods, institute some techniques of behavioural modification. Remember, habits that we have had since childhood will not be unlearned overnight. Occasionally, you may lapse into an old habit, particularly during periods of stress or pressure. Be aware that this may occur and take appropriate action.

Putting it together and assessing progress

So now that you have all the basic information — how do you put it together and assess your progress?

Gradually start implementing changes. Remember, your attack on your weight problem should be on three fronts — your diet, your level of activity and your habits with food. If it takes a while to get it all together, do not be discouraged. If your expectations are too unrealistic, you are setting yourself up to be disappointed. It is helpful to record in a diary the eating patterns which show your strong and weak points. In the diary, also record your level of physical activity.

Assess your progress both by objective and subjective means. Objectively measure your progress by weighing yourself once a week. Daily weighings are unnecessary and may result in frustration as weight tends to fluctuate from day-to-day.

Remember, scales measure total body weight. Total body weight is composed not only of fat but also fluid, muscle, bone and all the organs of the body. Up to 60 per cent of body weight is water. Undue emphasis on scales as indicators of your fat loss may confuse you. For instance, if you undertake a form of exercise that develops muscle (swimming or bike riding), the scales may show no weight loss because muscle is heavier than fat.

Therefore, do not focus on a set of scales as the sole indicator of your success when attempting to lose weight. Concentrate instead on subjective changes that will occur. Some of those changes are subtle.

Almost immediately after establishing a more sensible eating routine, you will feel more energetic. The less energy the body must expend in digestion, the more energy resources are available in other areas. You may notice it is easier to get up in the morning. You may sleep better. Indigestion symptoms will disappear. You will not get breathless on exertion.

As you lose weight your clothes will become more comfortable. Your self esteem will improve because you are confronting a problem and solving it. This will have a positive flow on to other areas of your life.

If you have a large amount of weight to lose, it is particularly important *not* to set an unrealistic target for yourself. Instead, set short-term achievable goals; these goals need not involve your weight at all. For instance; first, your goals may be to increase your level of physical activity by doing 20 minutes walking each day; to walk a flight of stairs without puffing; to develop a healthy cooking repertoire of recipes; to eat meals *only* when seated at a table, or to handle a stressful situation *without* resorting to food.

Once achieving your short-term goal, reward yourself (*not* with a high kilojoule snack), and then set yourself another short-term goal.

Once having attained a body weight with which you feel comfortable, continue to practise your new habits. Be on your guard against becoming complacent. Having lost excess weight, you can forget how bad that extra weight made you feel.

Do not try to hide if you feel you are regaining some weight. *Do not* avoid getting on the scales. *Never* resign yourself to buy the next size up in clothes because they are getting tighter.

Take a cool, objective look at yourself and try to determine in what ways you may have strayed, and how you can act positively to rectify the situation.

The benefits that a healthy diet and exercise regime have on your mind and body more than justify the self control that must be maintained in order to gain these benefits.

PUBLISHER'S NOTE

For further information about the 'Life. Be In It' Weight Management Centres — phone (03) 241 0333.

How to start the healthy diet plan

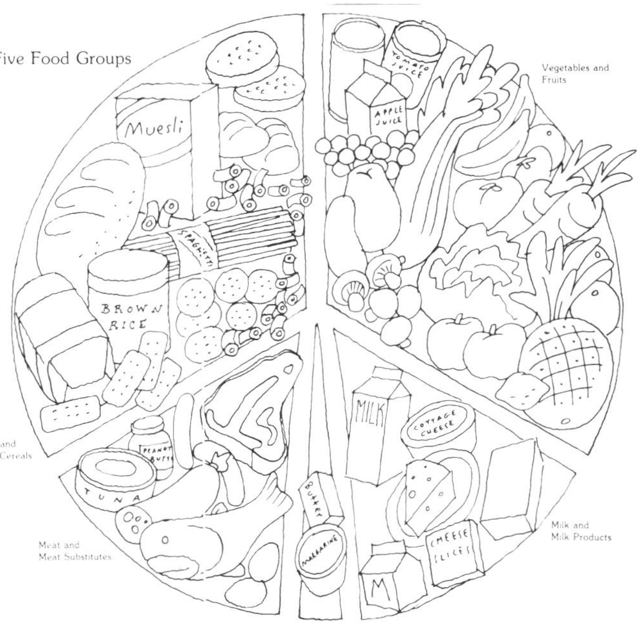

The More, or Less Diet has briefly introduced the foods we should eat *more* of, and those of which we should eat *less*. These foods form the foundation of the five food groups essential to a well-balanced diet.

Eat less fat

The body needs some fat because certain vitamins — A,D,E and K, which are only present in fatty foods — protect the internal organs and provide the body with energy.

However, we only require a moderate amount of fat. An over supply can result in overweight and obesity, and increases the risk of heart disease and some cancers.

Recent studies indicate that fat contributes more than 40 per cent of the food energy in the Australian diet. An upper limit of only 35 per cent is recommended.

Ways to help you eat less fat:

- choose leaner cuts of meat
- try the new milks, low fat

- buy yoghurt to replace sour cream
- try cottage cheese, low fat
- limit purchases of snack foods, such as potato chips, which have been processed in oil
- if tempted to buy pastries, cream cakes and other rich bakery goods and chocolates, remember, these are high in fat
- try desserts, sherbets, frozen yoghurt and fruit, low in fat
- if eating out at a restaurant or buying 'take-away' food, avoid fried foods, fatty mayonnaise and salad dressings

When eating:

- spread butter or margarine very thinly on bread or toast
- cut down on rich salad dressings
- cut any fat from meat before eating
- do not add butter or margarine to vegetables at the table
- cut down on rich gravies and cream sauces
- have rich cakes, pastries and desserts as an occasional treat — not on a regular basis
- have fresh fruit in season for desserts
- use plain or vanilla yoghurt as a dessert topping

Remember: moderation is important

Many foods which contain fat, also provide essential nutrients such as proteins, vitamins and minerals.

These foods include milk and milk products, meat, poultry, eggs, butter and table margarine, but they are necessary in the diet.

So, to obtain important nutrients without too much fat, use these foods in moderation and include some products low in fat.

Eat less sugar

Australia has one of the highest sugar consumptions in the world.

On average, about 1 kilogram of sugar, per person, per week, is eaten.

Large amounts of sugar in the diet can create problems because sugary foods often displace the more nutritious foods needed to provide vitamins and minerals. A high sugar intake also contributes to dental problems and overweight. Sugar includes brown and raw sugars, glucose, honey, molasses and syrups. Australians eat most of their sugars as refined sugars, (sucrose).

Ways to help you eat less sugar

When buying food:

- limit foods that are high in sugar, e.g., soft drinks, confectionery, cakes, pastries and desserts
- choose fresh fruits or fruits canned in fruit juice — not syrup
- read ingredient labels to check if added sugars are a major ingredient. In packaged foods, the ingredients are listed in descending order of concentration

When eating:

- add less sugar to foods such as tea, coffee and breakfast cereals
- reduce your intake of soft drinks, cordials and all other sweetened beverages
- choose fewer foods which are rich in sugar, such as cakes, biscuits and confectionery
- select fresh fruit in place of a rich dessert
- use less of all sugars, including brown and white sugar, honey, syrups and jams

Eat less salt

Salt (sodium chloride), is the major source of sodium in our diet. A small amount is essential, but most Australians eat much more sodium than they need.

Reduction of intake wherever possible is necessary; particularly for people with high blood pressure (hypertension). Avoid food with mono-sodium glutamate and soy sauce, high in salt. Food contains sodium naturally but much of the sodium eaten comes from salt which has been added to food.

Ways to help you eat less salt

When buying food:

- select low or reduced salt products, particularly bread, butter or margarine
- choose fresh vegetables
- limit purchases of foods to which large amounts of salt have been added; salted meats and fish, ham, bacon, corned beef, anchovies, smoked salmon, tuna in brine, and snack items; potato chips, salted nuts and crackers, bouillon cubes, cheeses (especially processed cheeses), canned vegetables, pickles and olives in brine

When preparing foods:

- do not use salt in cooking
- limit the use of other sodium sources, e.g., baking powder, monosodium glutamate and soy sauce, high in salt
- experiment with spices and herbs as seasonings

When eating:

- do not add salt at the table
- limit commercial condiments such as tomato sauce and soy sauce unless salt is reduced

Drink less alcohol

Alcoholic beverages are high in energy value but contribute few nutrients. Taken in moderation (1 or 2 drinks each day), many people find that alcohol contributes to their enjoyment of a meal or other social occasion. However, excessive drinking should be avoided as it can lead to nutritional deficiencies and diseases such as cirrhosis of the liver and some cancers, particularly if associated with smoking.

Drinking during pregnancy is not advised as it can harm the baby. Where weight control or reduction is desired, alcohol is high in energy and may be stored as fat. Therefore, either avoid or limit intake. Beers low in alcohol are preferable not only for the drinking driver, but for the health conscious. They are lower in kilojoules (calories) than standard beers.

Remember: it is acceptable not to drink alcohol

Food energey values for some alcoholic drinks:

1 can of standard beer (average 3.8% w/v alcohol)
(375ml) = 550 kilojoules 135 (calories)
1 can of low alcohol beer (average 2.4% w/v alcohol)
(375 ml) = 400 kilojoules (95 calories)
1 glass of wine (average 9.5% w/v alcohol)
(120 ml) = 400 kilojoules (95 calories)
1 glass of port/sherry (average 15.6 w/v alcohol)
(60 ml) = 350 kilojoules (85 calories)
1 nip of spirits (average 32% w/v alcohol)
(30 ml) = 270 kilojoules (65 calories)

Eat more breads and cereals

Breads and other cereals such as rice, pasta and breakfast cereals provide carbohydrate in the form of starch or complex carbohydrates — as well as food energy, protein and the B group of vitamins.

Their dietary fibre content aids the digestive system, which, in turn, reduces constipation and bowel problems. Wholegrain breads and other cereals contain more fibre, vitamins and minerals than refined products, so try to include wholegrain breads, brown rice, wholemeal spaghetti and noodles in the diet, rather than white breads and highly processed cereals.

Eat more vegetables and fruits

Vegetables are an important source of vitamins, minerals and dietary fibre; particularly the A and C group. These are some of the vitamin C vegetables:

Broccoli
Brussels sprouts
Cabbage
Cauliflower
Green peppers
Silver beet
Tomatoes

Some vitamin A vegetables:

Carrots
Tomatoes

Fruits also provide vitamins, minerals and dietary fibre — they are delicious as well as nutritious.

Some vitamin C fruits:

Oranges
Grapefruit
Lemons
Kiwi fruit

Balance the diet

Watch the amounts of food you eat, so that a healthy weight range can be maintained. If you are on a weight reduction diet, you may need more food than that which is included in the healthy diet plan.

Additional foods can come from the diet plan or you can include moderate amounts not specified, such as confectionery, cakes, biscuits and soft drinks. However, they should make only a minor contribution to the diet, the major share being selected from foods in the healthy diet plan.

Glossary for overseas readers:

agar agar	seaweed gelatine
beetroot	beets
capsicum	bell pepper
carob	St John's bread
cornflour	cornstarch
eggplant	aubergine

chick-peas	garbanzo beans
kiwi fruit	Chinese gooseberries
scone	biscuit
silver beet	use Swiss chard
snow peas	Chinese pea pods, mangetout
spring onions	scallions
pumpkin, butternut	winter squash
sultanas	raisins
sweet potato	yams, kumar
wholemeal	wholewheat
wholemeal, plain	all-purpose wholewheat
wholemeal, self raising	wholewheat self raising flour
zucchini	courgette

An explanation of some of the ingredients I use:

Chick-peas: are small, slightly rounded pulses, about the size of a pea. They are extremely hard and usually require soaking before they are cooked. Chick-peas are now available dry roasted and canned.

Low fat cheese: a range of hard cheeses, low in fat, suitable for grating. Carefully search the supermarket and health store shelves for the many different brands. Some varieties are less in salt content.

Nonfat yoghurt: most of the fat has been removed but not the calcium content. Use in cooking, dressings for salads, and, by adding apple juice concentrate, make a delicious topping for desserts.

Olive oil: the oil derived from olives. It is widely used in the Mediterranean countries and studies appear to suggest there is less risk of developing heart disease if olive oil is used where oil is recommended. It is mono-unsaturated and tends not to elevate either cholesterol or blood fat levels.

Parmesan cheese: a strong flavoured Italian cheese. Use only very small amounts grated, as a topping.

Filo pastry: very thin sheets of pastry stacked one on top of the other. Each sheet is often brushed with nonfat yoghurt or skim milk before use. It is available fresh or frozen and made from either white or wholemeal flour.

Ricotta cheese (low fat): a soft, unsalted, white cheese originally from Italy and used as a substitute for soft cheeses, high in fat. Although most of the fat is removed, it still retains calcium.

Tahini: a pale creamy paste which is the result of grinding sesame seeds together. It is used sparingly, because it is high in fat, but it does add that little extra flavour to the recipe.

Tamari or soy sauce, low in salt: a dark brown liquid, traditionally brewed from soy beans. The salt content is reduced and is suitable to use in recipes where a savoury flavour is desired. Those who are being treated for high blood pressure may need to avoid it altogether.

Weights and measures guide

This book uses standard metric weight and fluid measurements. It is always a good idea to have a reliable set of scales in the kitchen, *plus* a set of graduated cup and spoon measures.

The Australian Standard Metric cup is 250 ml.
The Australian Standard Metric tablespoon is 20 ml.
The Australian Standard Metric teaspoon is 5 ml.

Metric conversion

Dry measures

Metric: grams	Imperial: ounces
15 g	½ oz
30 g	1 oz
60 g	2 oz
90 g	3 oz
125 g	4 oz = ¼lb
185 g	6 oz
250 g	8 oz = ½lb
375 g	12 oz = ¾lb
500 g	16 oz = 1lb
750 g	24 oz = 1½lb
1000 g = 1 kg	32 oz = 2lb
1500 g = 1.5 kg	48 oz = 3lb
2000 g = 2 kg	64 oz = 4lb

Liquid measurements

Metric	Volume	Imperial
30 ml	1½ tablespoons	1 fl oz
60 ml	¼ cup	2 fl oz
90 ml	⅓ cup	3 fl oz
125 ml	½ cup	4 fl oz = US ¼pt
150 ml	¾ cup	5 fl oz = Imp ¼pt
250 ml	1 cup	8 fl oz = US ½pt
300 ml	1¼ cups	10 fl oz = Imp ½pt
375 ml	1½ cups	12 fl oz
440 ml	1¾ cups	14 fl oz

500 ml	2 cups	16 fl oz = US 1pt
625 ml	2½ cups	20 fl oz = Imp 1pt
1000 ml = litre	4 cups	32 fl oz

Oven temperatures

For successful cooking results, it is recommended that you use all Metric or all Imperial measurements. This will ensure success each time.

Celcius C	Farenheit F
120°C	220°C
130°C	250°C
140°C	275°C
150°C	300°C
170°C	325°C
180°C	350°C
190°C	375°C
200°C	400°C
220°C	425°C
230°C	450°C
240°C	475°C

Abbreviations

cal calorie
cm centimetre
g gram
kg kilogram
kJ kilojoule
in inch
ml millilitre
fl oz fluid ounce
oz ounce
qt quart
SR self raising

Preparing beans. Carefully examine the beans and remove any which are discoloured. Place them in a bowl filled with cold water. Remove any beans that float. Repeat this process several times until the beans are well washed. Soak them overnight before using and, to retain the water-soluble vitamins, use the water in the cooking.

Measuring beans. Use 1 part beans to 3 parts water.

Beans are full of vitamins, minerals and protein and can be included in a diet either as a replacement for meat or as an accompaniment.

To sauté onions. There is no need to use fat or oil. Place the onions in a nonstick pan. Heat, and add a small quantity of fresh vegetable juice, defatted stock or water. Cover, and gently toss as the onions begin to brown. You may need a fairly hot pan. Continue to cook for about 10–15 minutes until brown and soft. Add a little tamari or soy sauce, low in salt, if desired.

Stir 'fry' without fat or oil. Use either a wok or a nonstick pan. Heat and add the ingredients to be cooked. Toss with a little fresh fruit juice, defatted stock or water. Continue tossing as the ingredients cook.

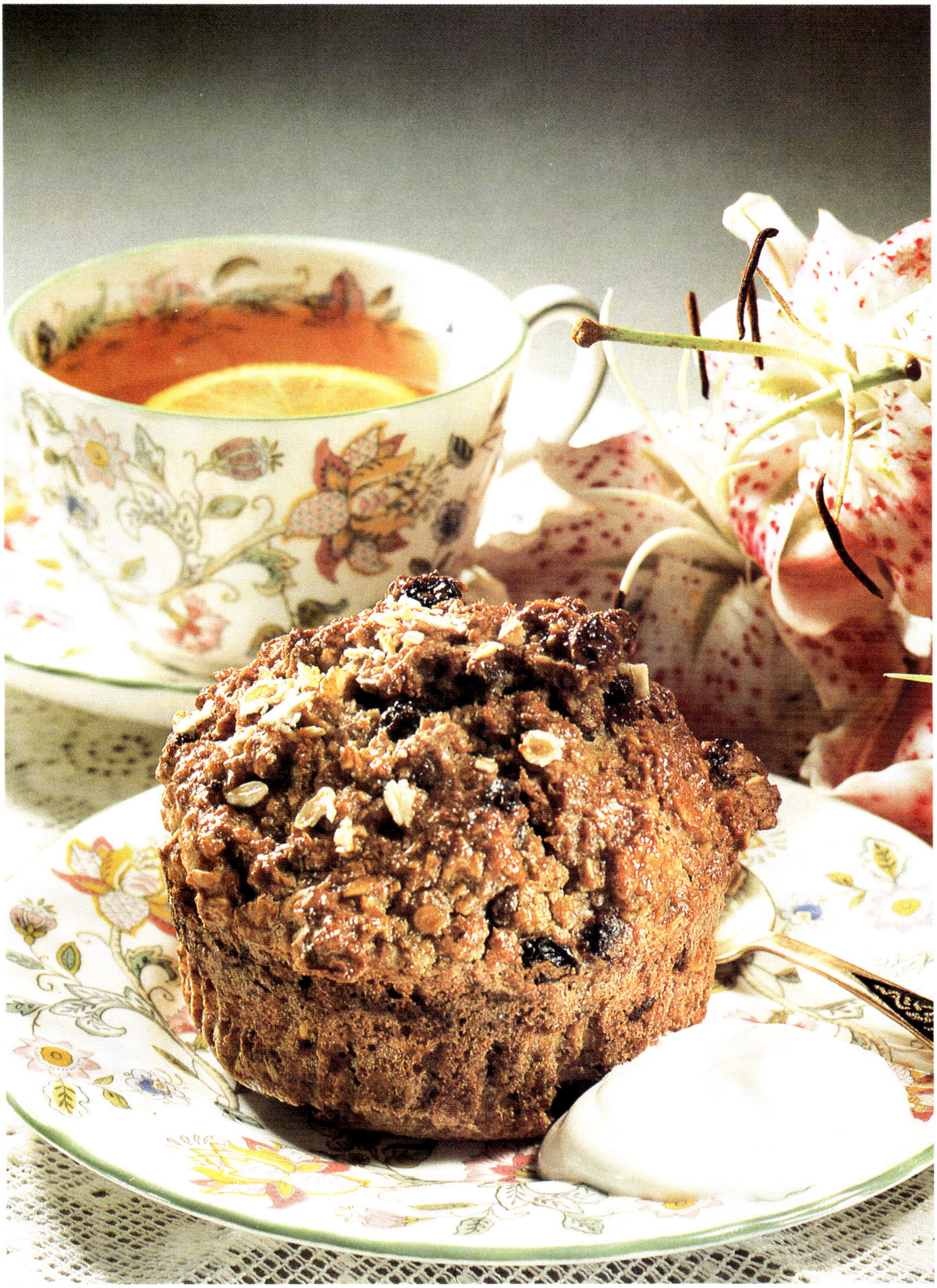

Oatbran muffins (*page 89*)
Vanilla ricotta sauce (*page 78*)

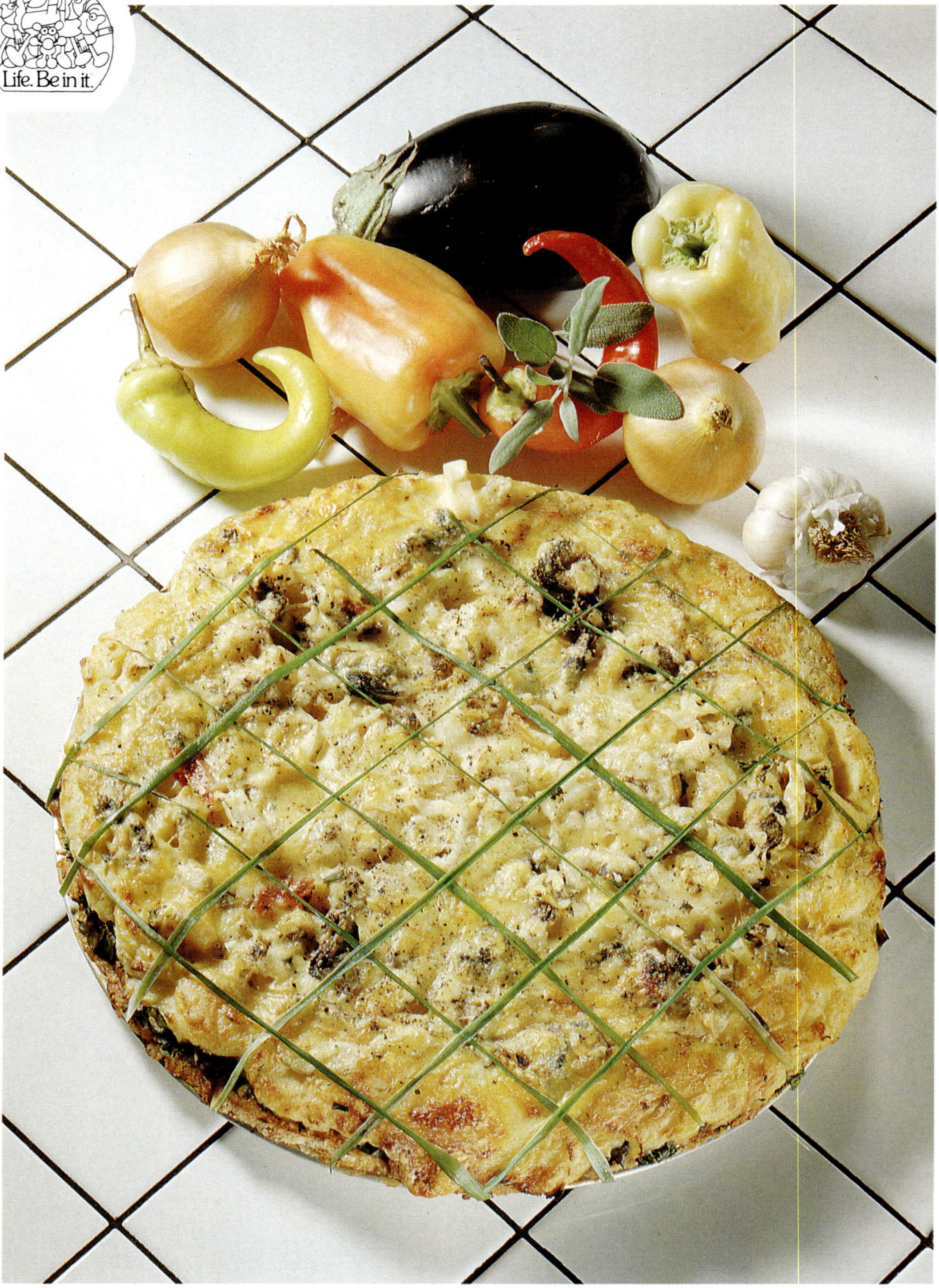

Seafood pizza (*page 63*)

Fats

Recipes to help you reduce fat intake.

Remember: moderation is important.

When preparing food:

- cut off all fat from the meat before cooking
- grill, steam, dry bake or stew meat, fish and poultry: avoid frying foods
- discard fat dripping from cooked meat
- chill meat and chicken soups, casseroles and stews until the fat becomes solid and remove it
- remove the fatty skin from chicken after baking
- season vegetables with herbs and spices instead of adding butter or table margarine
- use milk*, low in fat instead of regular milk in your recipes

Adding extra flavour.

The following are enhanced by many different herbs and spices. Here are a few selections you might like to use.

BEEF: allspice, basil, bayleaf, caraway, chilli powder, chives, curry, garlic, mace, marjoram, mustard, oregano, parsley, peppers (whole, pink and black), rosemary and thyme

CHICKEN: basil, bayleaf, garlic, marjoram, mustard, nutmeg, parsley, rosemary and sage

FISH: Bream — basil, coriander, dill, parsley, lemon and vinegar
Trevally — bayleaf, garlic, lemon, sage, thyme and vinegar

LAMB: dill, garlic, mace, marjoram, mint, parsley, rosemary and thyme

VEAL: basil, bayleaf, curry, garlic, marjoram, mustard, nutmeg, parsley, rosemary, sage and thyme

* Cheeses low in fat, nonfat yoghurt and skim milk are used and recommended in this cookbook.

Soups

Just imagine serving a thick hearty soup to the family on a cold night or a superb cold soup in warm weather. They may be successfully made without the addition of fat by using defatted stocks from beef, chicken, fish and vegetables, or water if you are in a hurry. Many ingredients including vegetables, grains, beans, pasta, rice etc. may be used to produce variety and provide nourishment.

Delicious soups may be served as an introduction to a dinner party or eaten as a meal, both in winter or summer with sandwiches. If you lead a busy lifestyle, make soups at night and refrigerate ready to use the next day. Hot soup can be taken to school or work in thermos flasks. The addition of herbs and spices will add flavour, particularly where salt intake has been reduced.

If you require a clear soup add a few egg shells for clarity. Remove them after several minutes.

Carefully skim the fat from soups and stocks.

Blended soups improve the flavour and consistency.

Simmer, *never boil*.

If a soup recipe requires wine, it is better to reduce the wine by half its volume to enhance the flavour. Parsnips, peppers, cabbage, are rarely added to stocks.

Stock

A good stock is the base of any good soup *or* sauce — whether it be chicken, meat, fish or vegetable stock. Freeze a few containers of stock — and a hearty delicious thick soup, or simply a broth with a few vegetables can be made in such a short time. There are no hard and fast rules for stock, just a little meat or fish and a few vegetables and herbs; boil for approximately 1 hour. Set aside to cool. Refrigerate overnight. Remove all fat. Put into storage containers and freeze.

Chicken stock

700 g–800 g chicken, bones, neck, breasts, chicken carcass etc.
1 large onion, sliced
1 large carrot, sliced
1 celery stalk
1½ litres water
1 bayleaf
2 sprigs parsley
¼ teaspoon thyme *or* 1 sprig fresh thyme
freshly ground pepper
dash of herb salt (optional)

Bring all ingredients to boil, cover and simmer approximately 1 hour. Cool, strain stock, refrigerate overnight. Remove all fat and place in containers and freeze if necessary.

variations

Vegetable stock

Recipe as above. Omit meat or chicken and add 1 leek (well washed), and sliced.

Lamb stock

Recipe as above. Use 1 lamb neck (fat trimmed), *or* 1 lamb shank. Alternatively, you may use 700 g of raw lamb bones, chopped.

Fish stock

1 large fish head *or* equivalent bones
1 onion, sliced
2 parsley stalks
1 celery stalk
4–5 cups water
½ cup white wine
3 peppercorns
1 bayleaf
wedge of lemon

Sweat the onion, celery and bayleaf for 3–4 minutes in a wok with a touch of oil. Place all the ingredients in a large saucepan and bring to the boil. Gently simmer for about 20 minutes. Skim the impurities off the top. Strain. Remove all fat collected on the surface. If not using immediately, this stock can be frozen.

Beetroot and broccoli broth

4 medium sized beetroot
1½ cups chicken stock *or* vegetable stock, recipe page 25 *or* water
1 bayleaf
1 cup broccoli flowerettes
1 tablespoon cider vinegar
¼ teaspoon nutmeg
freshly ground pepper
nonfat yoghurt (optional)

Wash beetroot well (removing all dirt), leave skin on and place in a medium size saucepan with stock and bayleaf. Bring to the boil, cover and simmer for approximately 45 minutes or until beetroot is cooked.

Remove beetroot (reserve cooking liquid), remove skin, purée in blender or food processor with 1 cup of cooking liquid. Add cider vinegar, nutmeg and season with a little ground pepper.

Steam or microwave broccoli until just tender and add to soup. If soup is too thick add a little extra stock or water. Serve with a spoonful of nonfat yoghurt, if desired.

Serves 4–6.

Chicken, rice and vegetable soup

For an even better taste: leave soup for 24 hours, then thin it down with a little stock, as the rice will thicken the soup overnight.

6 cups chicken *or* vegetable stock, recipe page 25 *or* water
1 large carrot, peeled and thinly sliced
1 large onion, chopped
1 celery stalk, chopped
½ cup brown rice, washed
1 cup chicken, diced (skin and fat removed)
fresh parsley, chopped
freshly ground pepper
pinch herb salt
1 bayleaf

Brush saucepan with a little light olive oil and gently sauté onion until soft. Add carrot, celery, bayleaf and stock with salt and bring to the boil. Add rice and simmer for 20–30 minutes until rice is cooked. Add chicken, a handful of chopped parsley, ground pepper, and simmer for a further 5 minutes and serve.

variation

Lamb, rice and vegetable soup

Recipe as above. Replace chicken with 1 cup diced, cold, lean, cooked roast lamb. Add to soup last and simply reheat. Do not recook as meat will toughen.

Serves 4–6.

Cabbage and bean soup

2 litres chicken *or* vegetable stock, recipe page 25
1 cup white navy beans, soaked overnight *or* for one hour in hot water
1 large onion, chopped
3 rashers chopped bacon — optional (rind and fat removed)
4 very ripe tomatoes, skinned *or* one can of tomatoes with the juice
¼ cabbage, shredded
¼ teaspoon ground cloves *or* 3–4 whole cloves
¼ teaspoon oregano
freshly ground black pepper
½ cup fresh parsley, chopped

Brush base of saucepan with a little olive oil and gently sauté onion and bacon until soft. Add stock, bring to the boil and add drained white beans, cloves, oregano and black pepper and simmer for approximately 1 hour until beans are tender. Add tomatoes, cabbage and parsley and simmer for a further 15 minutes. More liquid can be added if soup is too thick, but make sure you retain the flavour and do not dilute too much. Serve hot, sprinkled with a little fresh parsley and warm herb bread.

Serves 4.

Carrot, orange and ginger soup

For dinner party presentation: garnish with fine strips of orange rind that have been rinsed and boiled. This is for colour only, not taste.

750 g carrots, grated
1 onion, chopped
1 litre chicken *or* vegetable stock, recipe page 25
1 clove garlic
1 cm piece of ginger root, peeled and chopped
freshly ground pepper
¼ teaspoon nutmeg
juice of 1 large *or* 2 small oranges
parsley
nonfat yoghurt (optional)

Brush base of saucepan with a little light olive oil. Sauté onion, garlic and ginger until soft. Add stock and carrots and simmer approximately 25 minutes. Purée soup in a blender and add orange juice, nutmeg and pepper to taste. When ready to serve, reheat, and if desired, a spoonful of nonfat yoghurt can be added with a sprig of parsley.

Serves 4–6

'Cream' of cauliflower soup

¼ cauliflower head, chopped
4 medium potatoes, peeled and chopped
2 onions, chopped
1 leek, trimmed and chopped
2 celery stalks, chopped
6 cups chicken stock, recipe page 25
1 tablespoon tamari *or* soy sauce, low salt
bouquet garni, thyme, crushed peppercorns
pinch curry powder
pinch cayenne pepper
freshly ground pepper

garnish
few shakes of paprika

Sauté the onions, leeks, celery, bouquet garni and spices in a nonstick pan with a little stock until brown. Combine the onion mixture with the remaining ingredients in a large suacepan and gently simmer until the vegetables are tender. Purée them in a blender. Return the mixture to the saucepan and reheat, removing the bouquet garni. Top with the paprika and serve with crusty bread and a salad.

variation

Garlic 'cream' of cauliflower soup

Recipe as above. Add 1 or 2 whole cloves of garlic, crushed or chopped to the soup.

Cheesy 'cream' of cauliflower soup

Recipe as above. Add ¼ cup of grated cheese, low fat, about 10 minutes before serving. Garnish with 1 tablespoon parmesan cheese, freshly grated, and paprika.

Serves 4–6.

Life. Be in it.

Curried sweet potato and carrot soup

For extra flavour, add a squeeze of lime juice and a touch of nonfat yoghurt prior to serving this soup to your family or friends.

500 g carrots, peeled and chopped
3 large orange sweet potatoes
1 large onion, chopped
1 clove garlic, chopped
1 tomato, peeled
1 litre chicken *or* vegetable stock, recipe page 25
1 bayleaf
½ teaspoon curry powder
¼ teaspoon cumin
¼ teaspoon nutmeg
freshly ground pepper
pinch herb salt

Dry bake sweet potatoes on rack in hot oven until cooked, about 35–45 minutes, set aside. Brush saucepan with a little light olive oil and gently sauté onion, garlic, curry powder and cumin for a few minutes. Add stock, salt, chopped carrots and bayleaf. Bring to the boil and simmer for approximately 30 minutes. Remove bayleaf and purée soup in blender. Split sweet potatoes open and remove all orange potato flesh and add to soup. Reblend soup. Add nutmeg and freshly ground pepper to taste.

Serves 4.

Clear fish broth with prawns

To make this soup an attractive clear colour, add 2 egg shells and simmer for a further 5 minutes. Remove the shells before serving.

1 litre fish stock, recipe page 26
2 fillets fish (e.g., sea perch, John Dory boneless fillet)
500 g green prawns (cleaned, tailed and deveined)
½ teaspoon ground ginger
½ teaspoon coriander (ground)
½ cup red pepper, finely julienned (finely sliced)
½ cup spring onions, finely julienned (finely sliced)
freshly ground black pepper
fresh coriander

Bring stock to the boil, add ginger, coriander, red pepper and spring onions. Cut fish fillets into large bite-size pieces and add to stock together with prawns. When stock has reboiled, fish and prawns will only take 2 minutes to cook. Serve immediately with a sprig of fresh coriander in each bowl.

Serves 4–6.

'Fishestrone'

1½ litres fish stock, recipe page 26
1 large onion, finely chopped
3 rashers bacon — optional (rind and fat removed)
2 celery stalks, chopped
1 large carrot, peeled and sliced
1 tin tomatoes with juice (no salt), *or* 4 very ripe tomatoes, skinned
2 tablespoons tomato paste
½ cup cauliflower flowerettes
1 large clove garlic, finely chopped
3 fish fillets (boneless John Dory, sea perch *or* any white fish minus bones), chopped into chunks
1½ cups fresh seafood mix*
¼ teaspoon rosemary
¼ teaspoon basil
freshly ground pepper

Brush saucepan base with light olive oil. Gently sauté the onion and garlic until soft. Add bacon, carrot, cauliflower and celery. Stir 1 minute to prevent sticking. Add stock, tomatoes and tomato paste. Bring to boil and simmer 20 minutes. Add fish pieces, rosemary and basil and freshly ground pepper to taste. Simmer for a further 10 minutes. Serve hot with crusty wholemeal bread.

Serves 4.

* Seafood mix is now available from most supermarkets and fish shops. It contains scallops, calamari, shrimps etc.

Iced tomato soup with basil and chives

For a slightly different flavour, add half the quantity of wine with a bayleaf and some spring onions.

700 g ripe tomatoes, peeled
425 ml can tomato juice, unsweetened
3 spring onions
1 clove garlic
juice 2 oranges
juice 1 lime
fresh basil and chives
black pepper to taste
little white wine *or* mineral water
1 cup ice cubes

Chop spring onions and garlic in a food processor, add halved tomatoes and half of tomato juice. Process for 1 minute. Add remaining tomato juice, orange and lime juice, and black pepper to taste. Chill until ready to serve. Before serving, replace in blender with 1 cup of ice cubes and freshly chopped basil and chives: process for 1 minute. If desired, a little white wine or mineral water can be used to thin the soup.

Serves 4.

Minestrone

6 cups stock, recipe page 24, *or* water
2 potatoes peeled, diced
1 leek, washed and sliced
1 onion, chopped
1 large carrot, peeled and sliced
2 celery stalks, chopped
½ cup cauliflower flowerettes
2 leaves silver beet and stalks, washed and chopped, *or* spinach
2 large cloves garlic, finely chopped
3 rashers bacon (rind and fat removed)
¼ cabbage, shredded
¾ cup kidney beans, soaked in hot water overnight
2 tins tomatoes and juice, no salt *or* 1 large tin
2 tablespoons tomato paste
½ cup wholemeal macaroni
good handful chopped parsley
½ teaspoon basil
½ teaspoon rosemary
freshly ground pepper
pinch herb salt

Heat 1 tablespoon of light olive oil in a large saucepan and gently sauté onion, garlic, leek and bacon. Add stock, carrot, celery, kidney beans (drained), cauliflower and tomato paste. Stir well, bring to the boil and simmer for 20 minutes. Add the tins of tomatoes, parsley, basil, rosemary, cabbage, silver beet and potatoes. Reboil, add noodles and cook for a further 15 minutes or until noodles are ready. Season with freshly ground pepper.

Serves 4.

Mulligatawny soup

This recipe is traditionally served with cream, however, I suggest you use a little nonfat yoghurt. Curry and yoghurt are a great combination.

1 large carrot, chopped
1 onion, chopped
1 celery stalk, chopped
1 Granny Smith apple, peeled and diced
6 cups chicken *or* vegetable stock, recipe page 25 *or* water
½ cup nonfat yoghurt
¾ cup uncooked chicken, diced (skin and fat removed)*
½ cup brown rice†
freshly ground pepper
2 teaspoons curry powder
½ teaspoon cumin
¼ teaspoon thyme
good pinch herb salt

Brush saucepan base with light olive oil and gently sauté onion and curry powder. Add carrot and celery with stock and bring to the boil. Add rice, herb salt and simmer for 30 minutes until rice is cooked. Stir soup frequently, making sure rice does not stick to the base of the saucepan. Add apple, thyme, yoghurt, pepper and chicken and simmer for a further 10 minutes.

Serves 4.

* If you wish to use left-over cooked chicken in place of raw, simply add to soup at the final stage.

† Similarly, with left-over cooked rice, reduce cooking time for soup to 15 minutes then add the apple, thyme, yoghurt etc.

Pumpkin and apple soup

1 carrot, peeled and chopped
500 g pumpkin, peeled and chopped
1 large onion, chopped
1½ litres chicken *or* vegetable stock, recipe page 25
2 Granny Smith apples, peeled and chopped
1 ripe tomato, skinned and chopped
¼ teaspoon nutmeg
½ teaspoon curry powder
freshly ground pepper
freshly chopped chives
fresh dill, chopped (if available)
nonfat yoghurt (optional)
¼ teaspoon ginger

Brush saucepan base with light olive oil and gently sauté onion until soft. Add pumpkin, carrot, apple, tomato and stock. Bring to the boil and simmer 30–40 minutes. Purée soup through blender, add nutmeg, curry powder, ginger and ground pepper. Serve hot with a spoonful of nonfat yoghurt if desired, and sprinkle with chopped fresh dill and chives.

Serves 4.

variation
Add ¼ cup of apple juice concentrate for a stronger flavour.

Yoghurt is a good source of calcium. I use the nonfat variety for my recipes, to reduce the fat intake.

Vegetable and barley broth

1½ litres chicken *or* vegetable stock, recipe page 25
2 carrots, chopped
2 celery stalks, chopped
1 large onion, chopped
1 zucchini, chopped
1 small parsnip, chopped
½ cup cabbage, shredded and chopped
little broccoli and cauliflower stems, chopped
1 cup barley
fresh parsley
freshly ground pepper
pinch herb salt

Bring stock to the boil, add all chopped vegetables and barley. Simmer for approximately 45 minutes. Season with ground pepper, sprinkle with chopped parsley and serve with warm wholemeal bread.

Serves 4–6.

Zucchini soup

This recipe is the perfect **'Life. Be in it'** soup. You may add *more* or *less* of any of the ingredients and it will taste superb.

3 large *or* medium zucchini, sliced
1 onion, chopped
1 litre chicken *or* vegetable stock, recipe page 25 *or* water
¼ cup long grain rice
1 teaspoon curry powder
1 teaspoon Dijon mustard
pinch herb salt
½ cup nonfat yoghurt
freshly ground pepper
pinch herb salt

In a soup pot, gently sauté onion and curry powder in a little light olive oil. Add stock, rice, zucchini and herb salt. Bring to the boil and simmer for 15 minutes. Purée in blender, add the mustard and yoghurt with freshly ground pepper to taste. Serve hot or cold.

Serves 4.

Meats

Lean meat provides valuable nutrients that are required by the body to keep it healthy; these include protein and iron. It is also important to add a variety of lean meats to the family meals. Beef, veal, chicken, lamb, turkey *and* seafoods can be eaten on a regular basis, particularly where cholesterol levels are normal.

To ensure that the essential vitamins and minerals are included, alternate the meat recipes served to the family each week. Zinc, iron, niacin, riboflavin and vitamin B_{12} intake can be ensured by eating at least one red meat meal per week.

Of course, much research into the production of lean meat now sees a return to eating red meat, and sensible choices can be made when purchasing for the family.

Some useful tips to reduce fat intake when cooking meat

Roasting

Traditional Sunday roasts have long been favourite meals, and even though they are a source of increased fat intake, there is no reason why they need to be avoided.

To reduce fat in roasts:

- trim off all visible fat
- remove the skin
- cover the meat to be roasted with cabbage leaves *or* leek leaves (to keep the meat moist)
- roast meat on an oven rack
- add flavour by lightly painting the outside of the meat with soy sauce, low salt, and rubbing over with oatbran (this will form a skin)
- drain off fat as it collects
- liberally use stuffings, marinades, herbs and spices to add flavour

Sautéing or pan 'frying'

It is very easy to reduce fat intake by this method of cooking. The habit of using fat and oil in the pan is unnecessary and by making a few changes, quick meal preparation is assured.

- use a nonstick pan
- moisten the ingredients with vegetable stock *or* fresh fruit juices
- cover the pan with a lid to keep in the moisture
- use paper towelling to mop up any excess fat

Casseroles and stews

These are always appreciated by the family when the weather becomes cooler. For entertaining they can be prepared in advance; frozen, thawed and reheated. There is no limit to the variety of recipes using meat and vegetable combinations.

- trim off all fat and skin
- cut meat into small pieces, diced or in strips (for quick cooking)
- use water, defatted stock *or* fruit juice
- sauté meat in a nonstick pan first

Wok cooking

An excellent way of cooking to reduce both the fat intake and retain the natural vitamins and minerals in the food.

- trim off fat and skin
- cut meat into small pieces (for quick cooking)
- use shortcuts from the butcher
- stir 'fry' constantly to ensure the food will not stick
- use natural juices where liquid is required

Barbecuing

Barbecues are a traditional and accepted part of outdoor entertaining — in fact there is nothing quite like the smell of food being cooked on a barbecue. This is where crusty breads and a variety of salads can be eaten with a selection of cooked lean meats.

- use marinades, herbs and spices
- trim off all excess fat and skin
- use paper towelling to mop up excess fat
- cook meat in foil
- make beef *or* lamb shortcuts into kebabs
- introduce lean meats such as chicken fillets, marinated drumsticks (skin removed)
- be careful not to burn the meat
- make hamburgers or meat patties with lean minced meat; increase their size with oatbran and breadcrumbs
- brush meat with fruit juice *or* left-over marinade to keep it moist
- cook a wide variety of vegetables and fruit on the barbecue
- serve small meat portions with large vegetable servings

Beef, lamb, veal and rabbit

The following selection of red meats which I have chosen for your enjoyment, are very lean in saturated fats and dietary cholesterol.

Rabbit is extremely low and an excellent meat to add to your shopping list. Beef, lamb and veal are rich sources of iron which is necessary in a healthy diet.

When you remove the fat and skin from meat, particularly meats to be roasted, you may like to cover them with a glad bag, foil, or perhaps vegetable leaves e.g., leek, cabbage and spinach. This procedure will prevent the meat from drying whilst it is cooking.

Escallops of veal in lime and yoghurt

6 slices of veal
2 cloves garlic
plain flour
1 cup white wine
juice 1 lime *or* 1 lemon
2 tablespoons nonfat yoghurt (natural)
1 tablespoon fresh parsley, chopped
2 spring onions, finely chopped
freshly ground pepper

Ask your butcher to flatten the pieces of veal for you, or you can place the veal slices in between glad wrap and flatten it well yourself. Rub each slice of veal on both sides with a peeled garlic clove. Coat lightly with flour. Heat a heavy based pan to hot with a light brushing of olive oil. Place each slice of veal, one at a time, in pan and cook each side for 1 minute on fairly high heat. You may need to brush lightly with oil after each slice has been sealed. Remove to a platter and cover with foil. Heat lighty brushed pan again, and add finely chopped garlic and cook 1 minute. Add spring onions, toss 1 minute, add white wine and lime/lemon juice and simmer until liquid is reduced by nearly half. Sprinkle parsley and a little ground pepper over the top. Stir in the yoghurt and place veal slices back in pan, heat 2–3 mins and serve.

Serve with rice, steamed potatoes and green salad.

Serves 6.

Herb crusted rack of lamb

3 racks of lamb (6 cutlets on each rack)
3 cups of soft wholegrain breadcumbs
½ teaspoon marjoram
¼ teaspoon thyme
½ cup chopped parsley
1 clove garlic, minced
1 tablespoon tahini
juice 1 lemon

Preheat oven to 200°C. Remove all fat from racks of lamb leaving just meat. Using a sharp knife, remove white membrane covering the fillet and strip this away also.

Combine breadcrumbs, tahini, garlic and herbs and press firmly on to the meat. Bake in a nonstick baking dish, crumbed side up for 30–40 minutes. Check for desired preference in meat cooking time. It may need a little longer if you prefer lamb well cooked. Serve with steamed vegetables and perhaps fresh tomato sauce, recipe page 75.

variation
For extra flavour, brush the lamb racks with a little apple juice concentrate during cooking, and just prior to serving. It gives an attractive glazed effect on the meat.

Serves 8.

Lamb kebabs with coriander and lime marinade

1 kg boneless lamb from the leg (cut into bite-size pieces)
10 small baby onions, peeled

marinade
¼ cup pure apple juice
¼ cup fresh lime juice
1 teaspoon curry powder
½ teaspoon coriander
1 clove garlic, finely minced
¼ teaspoon tumeric
1 teaspoon honey
¼ teaspoon cumin
1 tablespoon fruit chutney of choice
freshly ground pepper

Place cubed lamb in bowl or dish. Mix all ingredients for marinade and pour over the lamb. Marinate in refrigerator 6–8 hours or overnight. Drain lamb from marinade (reserve for cooking), and thread on to skewers, alternating with small onions. Place under grill or barbecue for approximately 10–15 minutes, basting with marinade and turning frequently. Thicken any of the marinade that is left over with a little cornflour and serve as a sauce.

variation

Beef kebabs

Recipe as above. Omit the lamb and use cubed beef. Thread a mixture of vegetables of choice on to the skewers. e.g., sliced onion, red and green peppers, mushrooms.

Serves 4–6.

Korean barbecued beef

6 slices 'eye' fillet, approximately 2.5 cm thick
sesame seeds, toasted

marinade
¼ cup tamari *or* soy sauce, low salt
2 cloves garlic, chopped and finely minced
1 large teaspoon fresh ginger, chopped
1 teaspoon sesame oil
1 teaspoon lemon juice
¼ cup shallots, finely chopped
1 tablespoon honey
freshly ground pepper

Place steaks in a shallow dish. Combine marinade ingredients and pour over steaks. Cover and marinate 6–8 hours or overnight in refrigerator, turning at least 3–4 times. Remove steaks from the marinade and, if barbecuing, cook on lightly oiled grill plate, brushing with marinade during cooking, until done to your taste. Finally, sprinkle with sesame seeds.

Serve with cold rice salad, recipe page 102, and chopped green salad or baked potatoes, skin on, with a spoonful of cottage cheese, low fat. Decorate with freshly chopped chives and dash of paprika.

Serves 6.

Meatballs

These make a great addition to a picnic basket.

1 kg lean, minced, beef
1 large brown onion, peeled and chopped
1 clove garlic, finely minced
½ cup grated carrot
½ cup fresh parsley, chopped
1 teaspoon tamari *or* soy sauce, low salt
1 egg white
freshly ground pepper
1 teaspoon curry powder
a little wholemeal flour and wheatgerm, for coating

Preheat oven to 200°C. Place all ingredients in a large bowl and mix well, using your hands. Shape into small-to-medium size balls. Coat the outside of meatballs lightly with a combination of ½ wholemeal flour and ½ wheatgerm. They can be cooked in a nonstick frypan or a pan lightly brushed with olive oil until ready. *Do not overcook*. If preferred, you can bake on a nonstick tray in the oven until just cooked.

Makes about 8, depending on size.

Roast boned sirloin beef

If sirloin is not available, use either scotch *or* 'eye' fillet.

Trim away most of the fat, then puncture the sirloin in several areas with a steel skewer, filling the holes with a clove of peeled garlic. Sprinkle with rosemary and coat ⅓ of the sirloin with Dijon mustard and ⅓ with black peppercorns. Cook for 15 minutes per 500 g. This should be served underdone. The residue juices should be reduced in a pan or saucepan with an equal amount of red wine and reduced by half the quantity. Add chopped parsley and place over the top of the finely sliced porterhouse. Serve with hot steamed vegetables and green beans.

Serve 2 slices per person.

Meat-vegetable loaf

400 g lean, minced, beef
1 carrot, peeled and grated
1 small onion, peeled and finely chopped
1 clove garlic, finely minced
¼ cup celery, grated *or* finely chopped
¼ cup cabbage, shredded
¼ cup fresh parsley, chopped
¼ teaspoon thyme
¼ teaspoon cumin
½ cup wholemeal breadcrumbs
1 egg
¼ cup natural fruit chutney
freshly ground pepper

Preheat oven to 200°C. Mix all ingredients in a large bowl using your hands and place in a nonstick loaf tin or lightly greased oven dish. Brush top with a little water and some extra fruit chutney. Bake 10 minutes, then turn heat down to 180°C for approximately 20 minutes. Remove from the oven and leave in tin for at least 15 minutes.

Serves 4.

Eating less fat
You may have already cut down on your added fat intake and think you are eating less. However, there is much 'hidden' fat in commercially prepared foods. Therefore, to ensure your intake is much less, carefully read the labels to ascertain the type of fat, and how much is in the food item.

Rabbit casserole with apricots

1 whole rabbit and liver
1 tablespoon plain flour
220 g dried apricots
¾ cup chicken *or* vegetable stock, recipe page 25, *or* water
1 small brown onion
sprig fresh thyme
1 tablespoon fresh parsley, chopped
freshly ground pepper

marinade
1 cup red *or* white wine
3 tablespoons cider vinegar
1 clove garlic, finely minced
1 bayleaf

Cut rabbit into large pieces, remove the liver and keep separately. Place rabbit pieces into a glass or porcelain bowl with marinade ingredients and leave in refrigerator 6–8 hours or overnight (reserve marinade). Place dried apricots in a little cold water for approximately 1 hour.

Remove rabbit from marinade, dry and lightly coat with a little plain flour. Brush a heavy casserole dish with light olive oil and brown rabbit pieces at medium heat. Add onion and cook 2 minutes, turning gently. Add stock, ¾ cup of marinade, thyme, parsley and bayleaf, then season with ground pepper. Heat until liquid comes to the boil, stir well, reduce heat and simmer covered, for 30 minutes. Bake in oven at 200°C or simmer on top of hot plate.

Cut liver in pieces and add to casserole with drained apricots. Stir, cook for a further 30 minutes, until rabbit is soft and tender.

Serve with noodles and crisp green salad.

Serves 4–6.

Roast leg of lamb with sweet vegetable and herb sauce

1 leg of lamb, approximately 1.4 kg
1 large clove garlic, finely chopped
2–3 sprigs of rosemary
¼ teaspoon thyme
¼ teaspoon oregano
3 onions, peeled and chopped
2 large carrots, peeled and chopped
2 large cooking apples, peeled and chopped
2 tablespoons sultanas
3 tomatoes, sliced
1 cup white wine
½ cup water
freshly ground pepper
nonfat yoghurt

Preheat oven to 180°C. Trim and remove all visible fat from leg of lamb. Mix all vegetables and spread in the base of a nonstick baking dish.

Brush lamb with yoghurt, sprinkle with herbs and place meat on top of the vegetables in a baking dish. Cook in oven, turning meat two or three times brushing with yoghurt each time, for approximately 45 minutes to 1 hour. Remove lamb from tray, cover with foil and set to one side.

To make the sauce, remove and drain fat from tray. Purée vegetables, add wine to baking tray, bring to the boil and reduce by half. Add puréed vegetables, 1 tablespoon nonfat yoghurt, meat juices from lamb (in foil), and, if necessary, a little cold water. Season with ground pepper and pour into a warm jug or gravy boat.

Serve with roast or steamed vegetables and a green salad.

Serve 2 sices per person.

Chicken and duck

'Game' meats, with the exception of chicken, are usually very high in both saturated fat and dietary cholesterol. However, I have included a duck and beetroot salad, but concentrated more on chicken which has less saturated fat and dietary cholesterol. These recipes are delicious, and the use of herbs, spices, marinades and fruits, greatly contribute to the flavour of the dish.

Chicken and pinenuts

This recipe is served with a lime and yoghurt sauce.

1 large fresh roasting chicken *or* 6 fresh chicken fillets (skin and fat removed)
a little plain flour, seasoned with paprika and freshly ground pepper
1 small onion, chopped
1 clove garlic, chopped
1 celery stalk, chopped

garnish
1 cup water
freshly chopped chives
½ cup toasted pinenuts

sauce
1 cup nonfat yoghurt
juice and rind of 1 fresh lime
pinch nutmeg

Cut whole chicken into pieces, remove skin and trim off all visible fat. If using fillets, cut into half. Lightly coat each piece of chicken with seasoned flour. Brush a heavy based casserole or saucepan with a little light olive oil and brown each piece of chicken until sealed on all sides. Remove and drain on a paper towel. Reheat saucepan, lightly brush again with oil and gently cook garlic, onion and celery until tender. Put chicken pieces back into pot with the cup of water. Cover and cook (turning frequently), until chicken is tender and ready.

While chicken is cooking you can make the sauce.

Mix all the ingredients, pour over chicken pieces on a serving platter and sprinkle with paprika and freshly chopped chives.

Serves 6–8.

Chicken, mustard and broccoli quiche (filo)

The quiche may be served either hot or cold. When cutting, always use a knife with a serrated edge. Reheat in a microwave oven.
Line a 20 cm × 8 cm tin with nonstick baking paper. Make sure it covers base and sides, and overlaps all round to assist in lifting quiche from the tin, once cooked.

1 quantity of filo pastry
(enough to line base and sides of tin — 4 layers)

filling
2 cooked chicken fillets (skin and fat removed)
1½ cups cooked broccoli *or* cauliflower flowerettes
1 small onion, chopped
½ cup chives, freshly chopped
2 tablespoons Dijon mustard
3 eggs
4 egg whites
½ teaspoon paprika
freshly ground pepper
½ cup parmesan cheese, freshly grated
1 cup evaporated skim milk
½ cup skim milk

Preheat oven to 180°C. Brush filo sheets with skim milk on both sides. Line base and sides of tin with layers of filo to overlap by about 5 cm. Cut chicken into bite-size pieces and place in base of quiche. Add broccoli pieces. Cook onion gently in a small pan brushed with light oil until cooked, then add to chicken and broccoli. Sprinkle with grated parmesan, paprika, pepper and chives. Whisk eggs and egg whites, add evaporated skim milk, skim milk and mustard. Mix and pour over chicken and vegetables. Sprinkle with a little extra parmesan cheese. Bring filo pastry from sides, partly to cover top of the quiche. Cover with foil and bake in the oven for approximately 1 hour 10 minutes until quiche is set — removing the foil 10 minutes prior to the cooking time, thus enabling the quiche to brown. Remove from oven and leave 5 minutes. Carefully raise quiche with overlapping paper and place on a plate. Serve with green salad.

Serves 4.

Chicken sesame brochettes (kebabs)

6 fresh chicken fillets (skin and fat removed)
¼ cup tamari *or* soy sauce, low salt
1 tablespoon light olive oil
½ cup white wine
1 spring onion, chopped
1 clove garlic, finely minced
toasted sesame seeds

Cut fillets of chicken into bite-size pieces and place in a bowl. Combine remaining ingredients and pour over chicken and marinate for at least 4–6 hours or overnight. Remove chicken from marinade and thread on to skewers. Cook on barbecue or under grill, basting with marinade during cooking. When cooked, roll in toasted sesame seeds. Serve with rice and spoon over with warmed marinade.

Serves 4–6.

Chicken Waldorf salad

3 chicken breasts (skin and fat removed), steamed *or* poached until tender: *do not overcook*
2 celery stalks, sliced diagonally
2 large Jonathon apples, peeled and dried
¾ cup walnuts, chopped

dressing
½ cup nonfat yoghurt
juice ½ fresh lemon *or* lime
freshly ground pepper
pinch herb salt

Slice chicken into thin strips. Add celery, spring onions, apples and walnuts. Combine dressing ingredients and mix through salad. When ready to serve, sprinkle lightly with paprika.

Serves 3.

Chicken with rice and vegetables

This is a beautiful casserole and can be converted into a soup the following day, simply by adding chicken stock. Recipe page 25.

1 large fresh roasting chicken *or* 6 chicken fillets
2 cups chicken stock *or* water
1 carrot, peeled and sliced
1 celery stalk, sliced
1 onion, chopped
1 clove garlic, finely chopped
1 can tomatoes and juice, low salt
½ teaspoon oregano
½ teaspoon thyme
1 bayleaf
1 cup brown rice
freshly ground pepper
pinch herb salt

Remove skin and fat from whole chicken and cut into pieces. If using fillets, cut into bite-size pieces. In a large heavy based saucepan, brushed with a little light olive oil, gently cook the garlic and onion until tender. Add carrot and celery; stir, then add tomatoes with juice, stock, oregano, thyme and bayleaf. Bring to the boil. Add chicken and rice, cover and simmer 30–35 minutes or until rice is cooked.

Serves 6.

Cold steamed chicken with orange–lime and ricotta sauce

Serve this refreshing dish for a cold buffet.
Cut the chives longways — it adds to the appearance.

6 fresh chicken fillets (skin and fat removed)
juice of 2 ripe, sweet, oranges
juice of 2 limes
1 cup fresh ricotta cheese, low fat
freshly snipped chives

Steam or gently poach chicken breasts in a little chicken stock until cooked. When cooled, cover with foil and refrigerate until required. Blend ricotta cheese with orange and lime juice and pour over chicken. Sprinkle with freshly snipped chives.

Serve with 2 salads of your choice.

Serves 6.

Minerals
The most important minerals required by the body are iron, potassium (salt), calcium, iodine and sodium (salt). Although these are esential, the body only requires small amounts.

Duck salad with baby beetroot and pears

1 whole cooked duck (skinned, boned and cut into pieces), *or*
4–6 cooked duck breasts (skin removed)
half cup walnuts, chopped
baby beetroot (freshly cooked *or* tinned)
fresh herbs
1 bowl mixed salad greens (butter lettuce, mignonnette lettuce etc.)
2 pears, cut into 4, and sliced lengthways
2 spring onions

pear dressing
1 tablespoon cider vinegar
1 tablespoon fresh lime juice
½ teaspoon fresh ginger, chopped
¼ teaspoon lime rind, grated
1 tablespoon light olive oil
½ ripe, peeled, pear
freshly ground pepper

Preheat oven to 180°C. Cook whole duck, or duck breasts by baking in oven in nonstick baking tray or steam until duck is tender. *Do not overcook*. Set aside to cool.

Break lettuce into pieces and arrange on serving platter or in a bowl. Arrange pear slices on top. Duck can be arrayed in pieces, large slices, or cut into thin strips and tied into small bundles with lightly steamed spring onion strips.

Arrange duck on top of pear and lettuce. Sprinkle with walnuts, and spoon dressing over or serve separately. Decorate with fresh herbs and a few baby beetroot.

variation
Recipe as above. Omit the pears, but make up the pear dressing and spoon over the duck and salad. Alternatively, omit the pears and the pear dressing.

Serves 4–6.

Ginger and tamari chicken

6 large fresh chicken fillets (skin and fat removed)
2 cloves garlic, finely chopped
1 large brown onion, finely chopped
1 dessertspoon fresh ginger, finely chopped
1 tablespoon honey *or* unsweetened apple juice concentrate
½ cup tamari *or* soy sauce, low salt
½ cup water
1 tablespoon fresh lemon juice
freshly ground pepper
toothpicks
nonfat yoghurt (optional)
watermelon balls

Preheat oven to 220°C. Roll up chicken fillets and secure with toothpicks. Brush with a little apple juice concentrate or nonfat yoghurt. Place in non-stick baking dish and sprinkle top of each fillet with a little garlic, ginger, onion and freshly ground pepper.

Mix tamari, lemon juice, honey and water and pour in base of baking dish with chicken. Bake in oven 30–40 minutes. Turn chicken regularly, and baste frequently with cooking liquid. Bake until chicken is just done. *Do not overcook*.

Decorate with fresh watermelon balls and thin strips of spring onion. Serve with rice or noodles and green salad.

If desired, you may like to marinate chicken in the liquid 6–8 hours, or overnight to absorb extra flavour.

Serves 6.

Grilled apricot ginger chicken

This dish is very simple to prepare and is a good standby to have marinating in the refrigerator as it keeps for up to 24 hours.

6 fresh chicken fillets (skin and fat removed)
½ cup water
1 clove garlic, finely chopped
1 cup dried apricots
1 teaspoon fresh ginger, finely chopped
1 spring onion, chopped
1 tablespoon nonfat yoghurt
¼ teaspoon cayenne pepper
juice 1 lemon *or* lime

Place apricots, lemon juice and water in small saucepan and bring to the boil. Gently simmer until tender; alternatively, this can be done in a microwave. Place in blender with garlic, spring onion, ginger, cayenne and yoghurt. Purée the ingredients. Place chicken fillets in shallow dish and make a few cuts in each one. Cover with apricot mixture and marinate in refrigerator for 3–4 hours or overnight. Place chicken on to a grill tray and brush with a little yoghurt. Grill slowly until tender. (Keep spooning apricot sauce over chicken during grilling).

Serve over boiled rice and perhaps a large green salad.

Serves 6.

Life. Be in it.

Indonesian peanut chicken

2 cups cold brown rice, cooked, recipe page 96
6 chicken fillets (skin and fat removed), steamed *or* poached in a little chicken stock until tender; cool and cut into bite-size pieces

peanut sauce
1 cup unsalted, peanuts, roasted and shelled
1 small brown onion
1 clove garlic
1 teaspoon fresh ginger, finely chopped
1 tablespoon tamari *or* soy sauce, low salt
1 teaspoon curry powder
1 teaspoon turmeric
1 cup water
juice 1 lime *or* lemon

Place all ingredients for sauce in blender or food processor and process until smooth. Gently simmer sauce until it thickens, approximately 15 minutes. Spoon rice on to serving platter and place chicken on top. Spoon peanut sauce over the chicken. Serve with one of the tempting salads in this book.

Serves 6.

Steamed chicken in avocado 'cream' sauce

The avocado sauce may be made into a dip. Add a pinch of curry powder for added flavour.

6 fresh chicken fillets (skin and fat removed)

avocado sauce
½ cup nonfat yoghurt
1 ripe avocado
½ cup plain cottage cheese, low fat
1 tablespoon fresh chives, chopped
1 teaspoon lemon juice
pinch cayenne pepper
freshly ground pepper

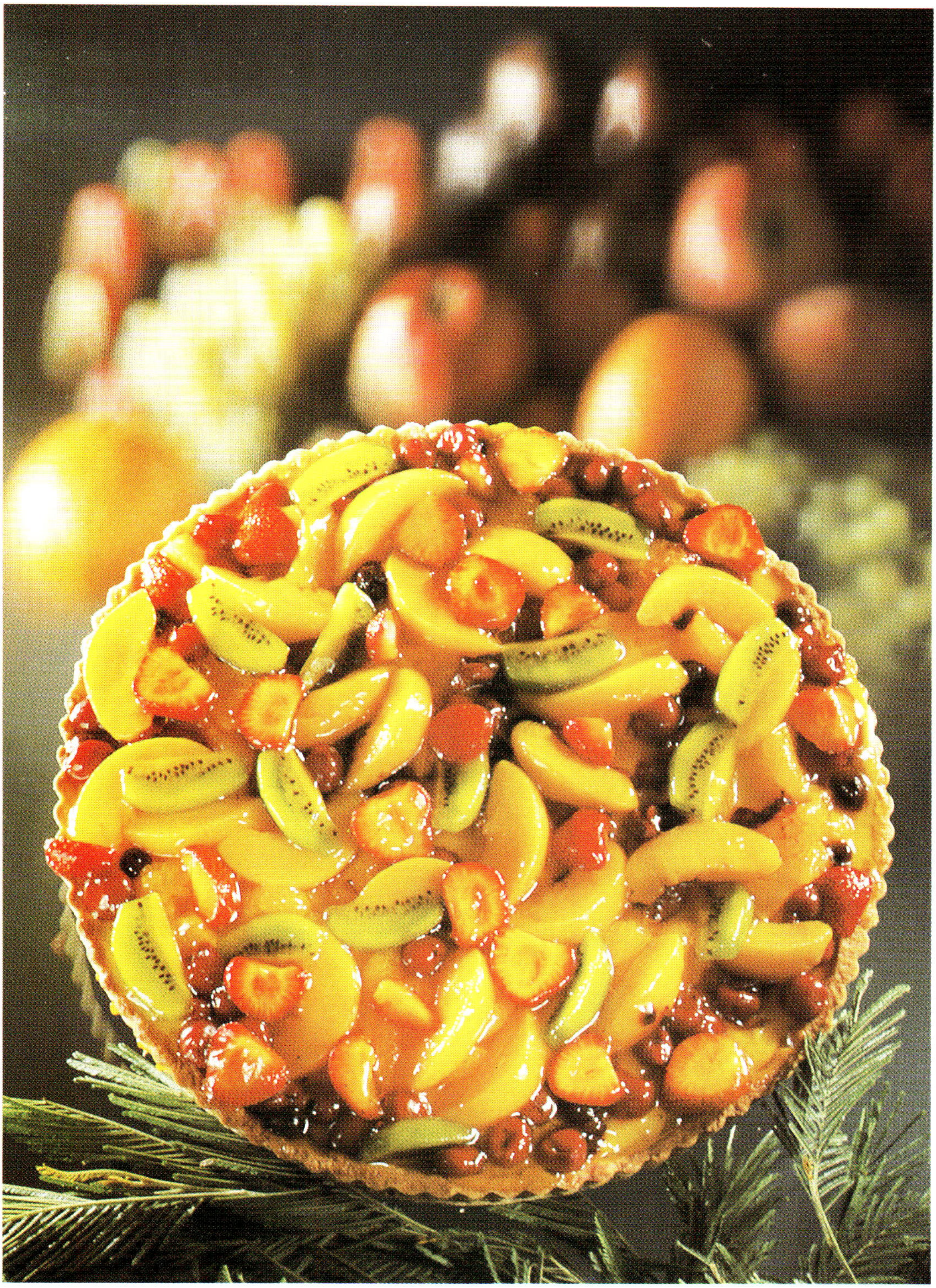

Mixed fruit flan (*page 88*)
Fruit glaze (*page 76*)

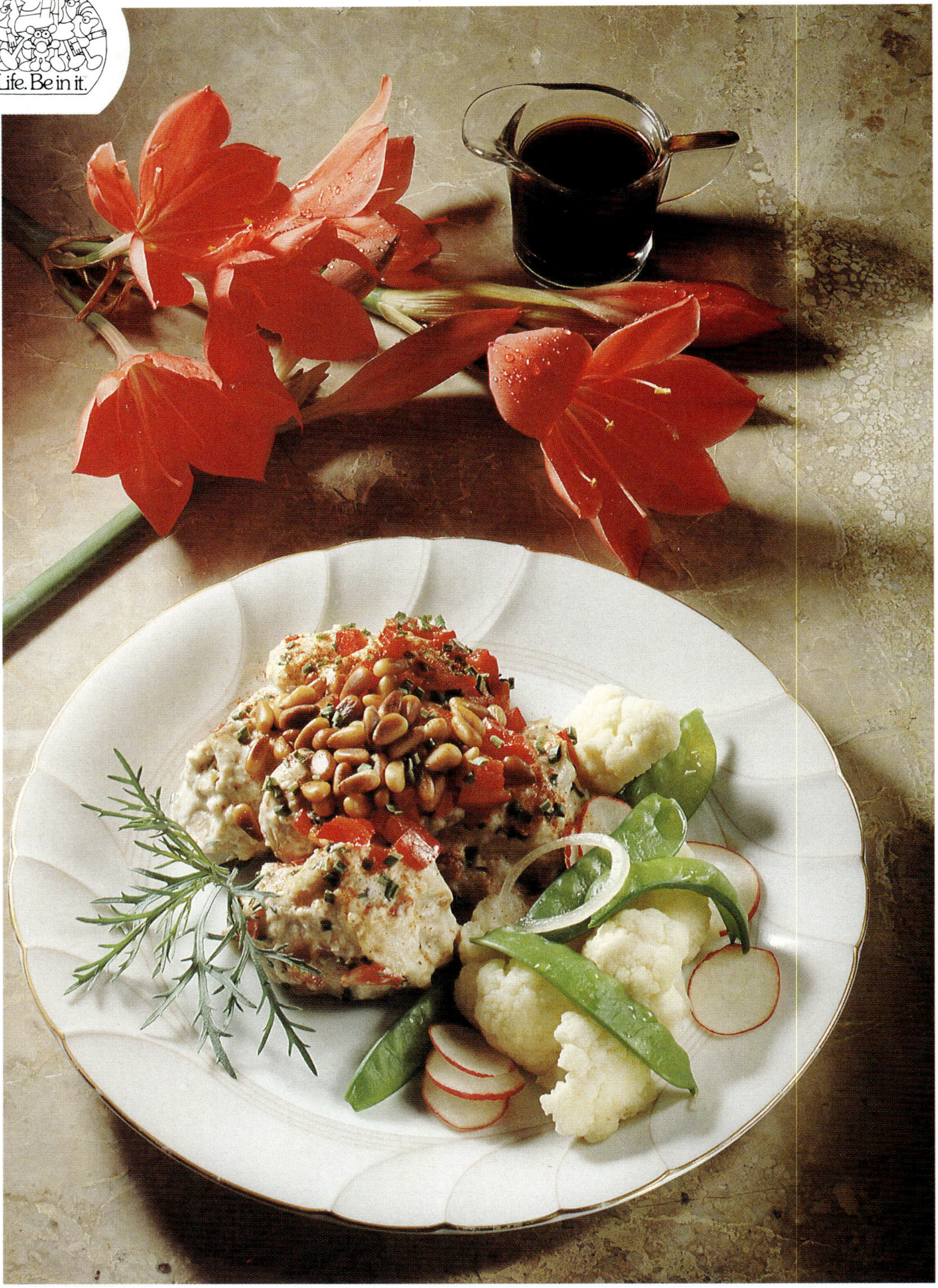

Chicken and pinenuts (*page 46*)
Cauliflower salad (*page 129*)

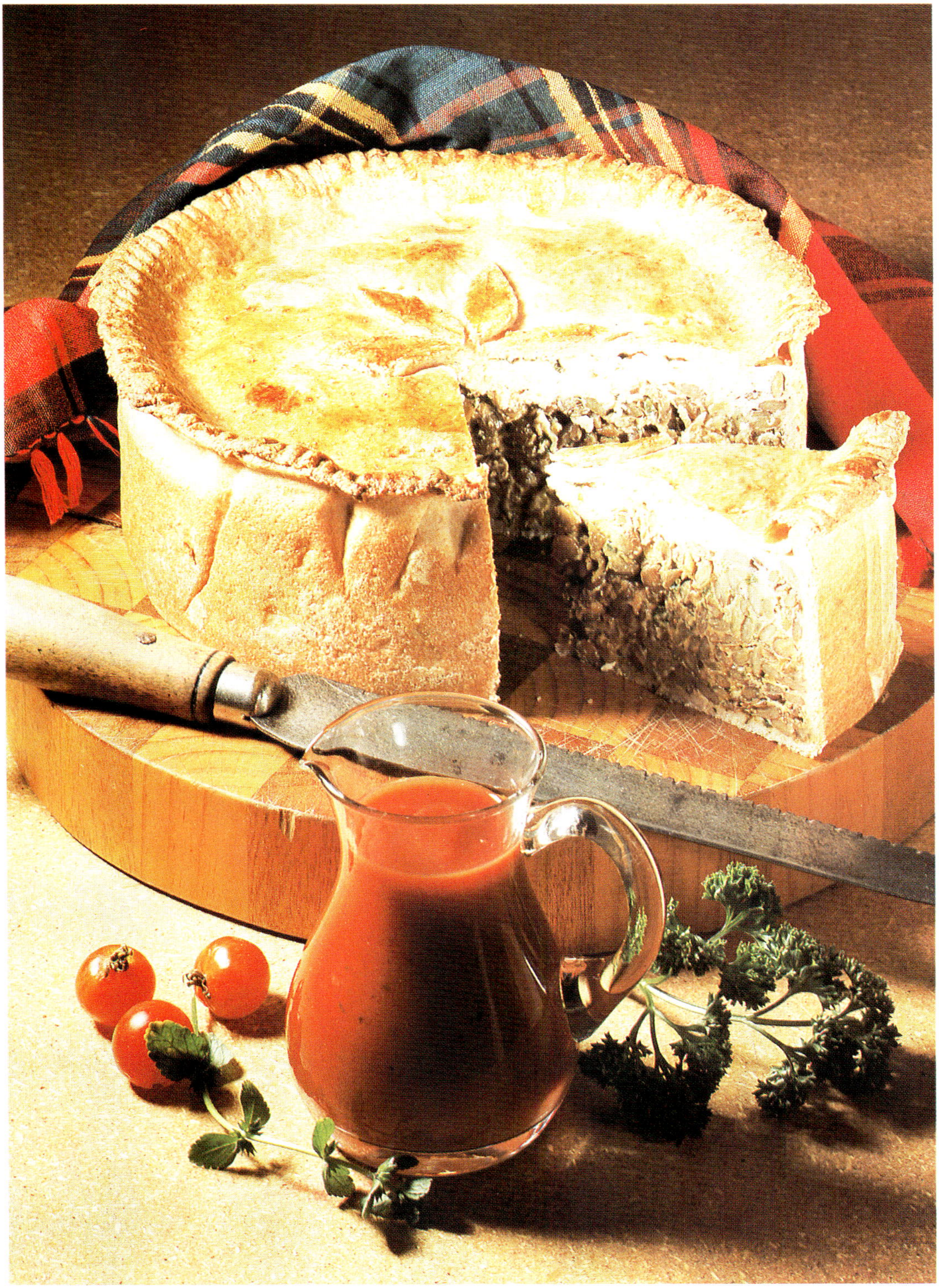

Lentil pie (*page 101*)
Fresh tomato sauce (*page 75*)

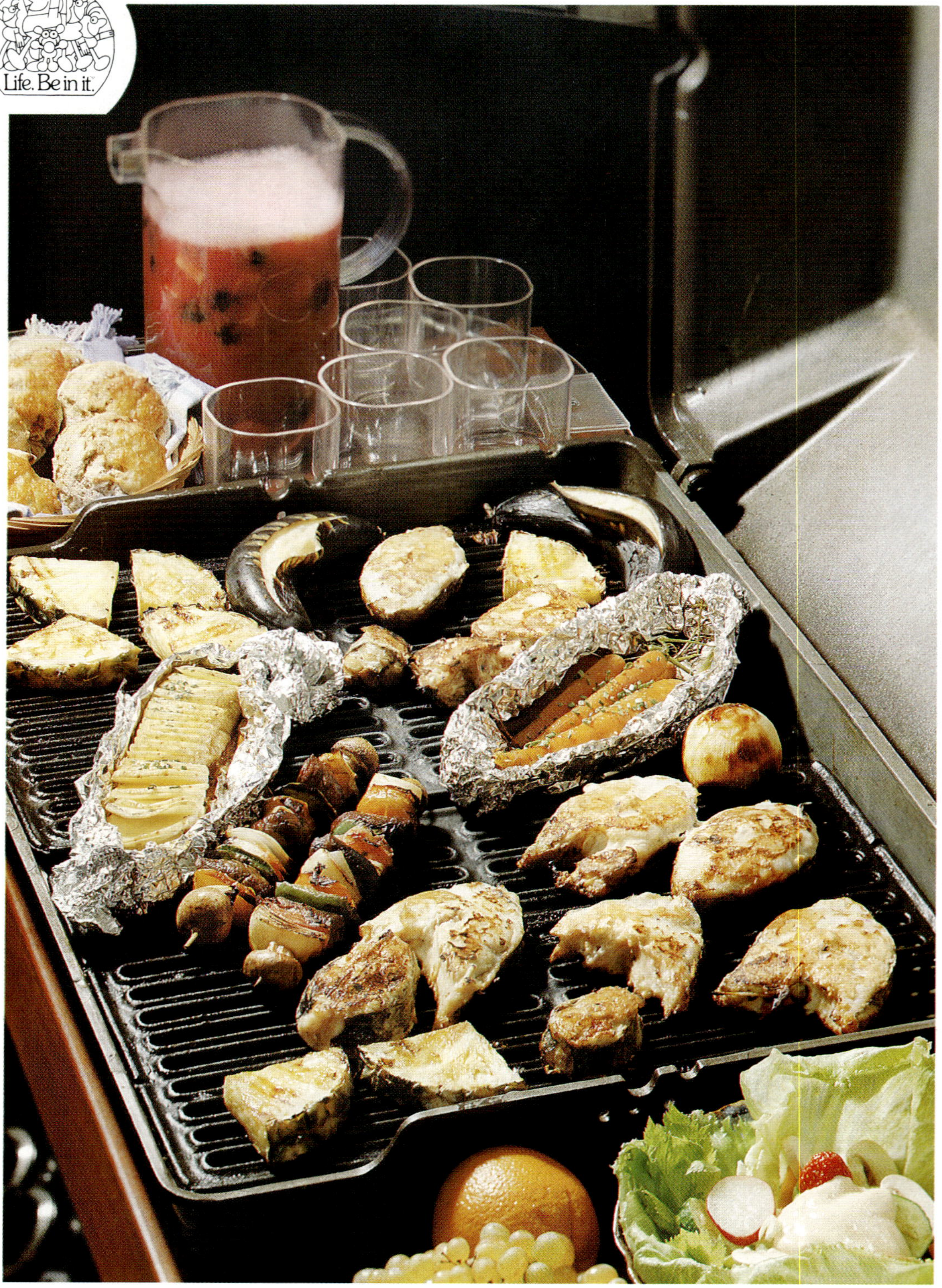

Barbecued pineapple (*page 135*), Barbecued potatoes (*page 110*) and carrots (*page 110*), Barbecued whole bananas (*page 135*), Fruit salad punch (*page 141*), Lime and yoghurt dressing (*page 77*), Marinated fish steaks (*page 62*), Tossed mixed salad (*page 132*), Wholemeal cheese scones (*page 94*),

Gently poach or steam chicken fillets until tender. Place on serving platter, cover with foil and keep warm. Purée all ingredients in blender and, when ready to serve, arrange chicken on platter and carefully pour sauce down the middle of each fillet. Sprinkle with the extra chopped chives.

Serve with a salad of your choice.

Serves 6.

Steamed whole chicken orange soy

Delightful the next day, served cold with a touch of herb salt.

1 large, fresh, roasting chicken
1 small brown onion, halved
½ cup chicken stock, recipe page 25
1 tablespoon tamari *or* soy sauce, low salt
juice of two large, sweet, oranges
1 dessertspoon unbleached white flour
1 teaspoon fresh ginger, finely chopped
¼ teaspoon Chinese five spices
freshly ground pepper
peel of 1 orange
a little chicken stock

Remove the skin and fat from the chicken, wash under cold water and pat dry. Put the orange juice, soy sauce, stock, ginger and spice in a saucepan. Add the onion and orange peel to the cavity of the chicken. Place the chicken into the saucepan with the liquids and bring to the boil. Gently simmer about 1 hour, occasionally spooning the liquid over the chicken. Arrange the cooked chicken on a serving platter and skim any fat from the top of the liquid. Thicken with the unbleached flour mixed with the extra stock. Serve over the chicken. This is absolutely delicious when served with steamed brown or 'fried' rice, or noodles and steamed broccoli.

Tandoori chicken

1 large, fresh, roasting chicken *or* 6 chicken fillets (skin and fat removed)
1 clove garlic, finely chopped
1 dessertspoon fresh ginger, grated *or* finely chopped
1 cup nonfat yoghurt
1 teaspoon curry powder
1 teaspoon Dijon mustard
1 tablespoon lemon juice
¼ teaspoon chilli powder
1 teaspoon paprika
¼ teaspoon coriander
¼ teaspoon freshly ground pepper

Cut whole chicken in portions. Make a few small cuts in chicken pieces to absorb flavour of marinade. Place garlic and ginger in blender or food processor and process for 2 seconds. Add all remaining ingredients, mix, and pour over chicken in shallow nonstick baking dish. Marinate in refrigerator 3–4 hours or overnight.

When ready to use, preheat the oven to 200°C. Place the chicken pieces on a tray covered with baking paper and dry bake in the oven or place under a grill until cooked. You can also barbecue the chicken pieces.

Serves 4–6.

Fish and seafood

You will really enjoy these fish and seafood recipes. Some will contain less saturated fat and dietary cholesterol than others. It is always a good idea to remove the skin from the fish *before* it is cooked. This will reduce much of the fat content in the recipe. There is now evidence that some oily fish may reduce blood clotting. I have used herbs, spices, fruit and vegetables to increase the fibre in these recipes as well as to enhance the flavour.

Baked dill fish

6 fresh fillets (medium size), e.g., John Dory, sea perch, trevally, rockling etc.
¼–½ cup fresh lime juice
1 clove garlic, crushed and finely minced
1 teaspoon dill
sprinkle of herb salt
freshly ground pepper

Place fillets of fish in a nonstick baking dish, cover with lime juice and garlic and sprinkle with herb salt and ground pepper. Marinate in refrigerator for 30 minutes before baking in a moderately hot oven for approximately 8–10 minutes. *Do not overcook*. Serve with a slice of lime, steamed baby potatoes and a tossed salad.

Serves 4–6.

Calamari and capsicum salad

When using and preparing calamari, a much better result will be achieved if you cut it finely. In this recipe the tubes (body), not the legs are preferred.

1 kg fresh calamari, cut into rings
½ green capsicum
½ red capsicum
1 red spanish onion, peeled and sliced
fresh parsley, chopped

dressing
1 tablespoon light olive oil
1 clove garlic, finely chopped
2 tablespoons grapefruit juice *or* lemon juice
dash herb salt
freshly ground pepper

Cook calamari in boiling water 3–4 minutes. Drain and arrange in salad bowl. Wash and seed capsicum and slice into thin strips. Add to bowl with onion and a handful of fresh chopped parsley. Mix dressing and pour over.

Serves 4–6.

Calamari with mushrooms, pasta and fresh tomato sauce

Calamari may be sautéd in a touch of olive oil in a hot pan for 2–3 minutes. Remember, the longer you cook calamari the tougher it becomes. Be careful: *do not overcook*.

500 g calamari, sliced into rings
300 g wholemeal pasta shells
1–1½ cups dry white wine
1 teaspoon lemon *or* lime juice
2 cups mushrooms, sliced
1 quantity fresh tomato sauce, recipe page 75
fresh basil, extra
1 tablespoon fresh chives, chopped
freshly ground pepper

Place pasta in boiling water until cooked: *do not overcook*, drain under cold water and set aside. Prepare 1 quantity of fresh tomato sauce. Put calamari in a large nonstick saucepan, cover with wine and limes or lemon juice and simmer until calamari is almost cooked, 3–5 minutes. Add fresh tomato sauce, mushrooms, chives, a little ground pepper, and pasta. Stir through and simmer for a further 5–8 minutes. Serve with extra basil leaves sprinkled on top.

Serves 4–6.

Fish curry

This dish may be garnished with either watermelon or cantaloup balls. For good presentation, use a melon baller.

6 fresh cutlets of fish (schnapper, trevally, jew fish), small to medium size
2 cloves garlic, chopped
3 large onions, peeled and sliced
1 tablespoon fresh ginger, chopped
3 red chillies (optional)
1 teaspoon turmeric
2 cups fish stock, recipe page 26, *or* water
1 tablespoon apple juice concentrate *or* 1 tablespoon honey
½ cup cider vinegar
1 bayleaf
1 teaspoon dried coriander
1 teaspoon cumin
1 teaspoon cloves
1 tablespoon curry powder

Brush a large heavy based pot with a little olive oil and heat. Gently sauté onions, garlic, ginger and seeded chillies until soft. Remove from pot with slotted spoon and set aside. Rebrush with oil, add tumeric, curry powder, cumin and cloves. Stir for a few minutes then add the fish. When fish is golden on both sides, add stock and return garlic, onion, ginger and chillies to pot. Add honey, vinegar and bayleaf. Bring to the boil, lower heat and simmer for approximately 20 minutes. If possible, cook any curry dish 12–24 hours before eating. Refrigerate, and reheat when ready to serve.

Serves 6.

Grilled cutlets *or* whole fish with ginger

If you decide to dry bake fish in the oven, it will not be necessary to turn the fish.

6 medium cutlets *or* fillets *or* small whole fish
½ cup plain flour, seasoned with herb salt and ground pepper
3 teaspoons freshly ground pepper
lemon juice *or* lime juice
freshly ground pepper (extra)

Brush a flat baking tray with a little light olive oil. Coat fish in seasoned flour and place on a baking tray, skin side up. Squeeze a little lemon or lime juice over the fish, sprinkle with freshly ground pepper and a dash of herb salt. Place under a hot grill for 3–5 minutes (according to size and thickness of fish). Turn carefully on to other side, sprinkle with ginger, a little more lemon or lime juice and another dash of pepper. Return under grill to cook other side.

Serve with lemon or lime wedges, whole baked potatoes and a salad from the salad section.

Serves 6.

Sesame seeds add a wonderful flavour, especially if they are dry baked or tossed in a nonstick pan until brown. When purëed in a blender, they are a delicious accompaniment to a salad.

Marinated fish steaks

The best results for cooking fish are achieved when the hot plate is at the correct temperature. It must be hot for pan 'frying', grilling or barbecuing. The fish does not cook as well if the hot plate is not at the right heat. Turn fish once only.

8–10 medium size cutlets of fish (e.g., trevally, schnapper)
1 tablespoon lemon juice *or* lime juice
¼ cup orange juice
1 clove garlic, chopped and finely minced
1 tablespoon chives, freshly chopped
¼ cup white wine
½ tablespoon oregano

Place fish steaks in a shallow dish. Mix marinade and pour over fish. Cover with cling wrap and marinate several hours or overnight in the refrigerator.

Fish steaks can be barbecued, cooked in a nonstick frypan, or in a pan lightly coated with olive oil, until golden and ready. Whichever way you choose, *do not overcook*.

Serves 8–10.

All fats and oils have the same amount of cal/kJ. I recommend using olive oil or polyunsaturated oil very sparingly when cooking.

Seafood pizza

A quantity of pizza 'sour' dough, recipe page 69
1 cup skim milk white sauce, recipe page 80
½ cup fresh tomato sauce, recipe page 75
1–1½ cups mixed, chopped seafood, e.g., scallops, prawns, shrimps, fish etc.
½ teaspoon basil
freshly ground pepper

topping
grated cheese, low fat

Preheat the oven to 220°C. Roll out the dough and cover a large pizza tray or 4 small trays. You may like to paint each tray with nonfat yoghurt first. Spread a layer of fresh tomato sauce over the dough and then the white sauce on top of the tomato sauce. Sprinkle with the chopped seafood, pour over a little tomato sauce, basil and ground pepper. Top with the grated cheese and bake in the oven about 15–30 minutes or until the pastry base is cooked.

Salmon 'burgers'

Another delicious addition to a picnic basket.

1 210 g canned salmon, pink *or* red
1 cup mashed potato
½ cup carrot, grated
1 small onion, finely chopped
1 egg white
¼ teaspoon nutmeg
¼ teaspoon curry powder
1 teaspoon lemon juice
freshly ground pepper

coating
wholemeal flour *or* oatbran

Mix all the ingredients by hand and shape into small or medium patties. Lightly coat each pattie with the flour or oatbran. Brown each side in a nonstick pan.

Makes about 4 patties.

Seafood salad supreme

500 g fresh scallops
1 kg fresh mussels, cleaned
750 g cooked prawns (cleaned, deveined and peeled)
300 g calamari, sliced into rings
1 onion, peeled and sliced
1 cup dry white wine
1–2 cups fish stock, recipe page 26 *or* water
¼ cup chives, chopped
¼ cup fresh parsley, chopped
dash herb salt
freshly ground pepper

Cook calamari in a large saucepan with white wine, onion and stock or water. Simmer gently until calamari is tender. Remove calamari with slotted spoon to a serving bowl and allow to cool. Add scallops to same liquid, cook 1–2 minutes, remove with slotted spoon to bowl containing the calamari. Add mussels to saucepan (make sure you have enough wine, if not, add a little more). Cook gently until mussels open. Remove from saucepan and cool. Take mussels from shells and add to calamari and scallops. Sprinkle with chopped chives and parsley.

dressing
1 tablespoon light olive oil
1 tablespoon lime *or* lemon juice
1 clove garlic, crushed and finely chopped
1 teaspoon Dijon mustard
freshly ground pepper

Pour over seafood mix and toss through. Refrigerate 2–3 hours and serve.

Serves 6–8.

Seafood crêpes

a quantity fresh tomato sauce, recipe page 75
6–8 wholemeal crêpes, recipe page 95
a quantity skim milk white sauce, recipe page 80
1 kg mixed seafood (fish pieces, calamari, scallops and prawns)
1½ cups white wine *or* 1½ cups fish stock, recipe page 26
1 tablespoon fresh lemon *or* lime juice
¼ cup fresh chives, chopped
¼ cup fresh parsley, chopped
½ teaspoon tarragon
½ teaspoon basil
½ teaspoon paprika
freshly ground pepper

Prepare crêpes as per recipe. Gently poach seafood mix in white wine or stock in nonstick saucepan and simmer until just cooked. Drain and set aside to cool. When cooled, add to white sauce with tarragon, basil, paprika, ground pepper and lemon juice. Stir through.

Divide mixture, by spooning into centre of each crêpe. Roll up carefully and place each crêpe in a shallow oblong pasta serving dish (which has been lightly greased), or nonstick baking dish. Pour fresh tomato sauce over top and bake in a moderately hot oven 25–30 minutes and serve. Alternatively, crêpes can be heated in a microwave and sauce served separately in a jug. This dish is also delicious served cold.

Serves 6–8.

Steamed fish with yoghurt and chive sauce

6 medium size fresh fish fillets (e.g., John Dory, sea perch)
yoghurt and chive sauce
1½ cups nonfat yoghurt
¼ cup fresh chives, chopped
1 tablespoon fresh parsley, chopped
¼ teaspoon fresh *or* dried coriander
dash herb salt
freshly ground pepper

Combine all ingredients for sauce. This may be served warm or cold.

Gently steam or microwave the fish for approximately 5–10 minutes (depending on size and texture of fish), 2 pieces at a time. Keep warm, sprinkle with lemon juice and a little chopped fresh coriander. Cover and keep warm in a preheated, just warm oven. When ready, sauce may be warmed and drizzled over fish or served in a separate jug. Serve with a chopped green salad, herb and sesame beans, or a selection of fresh steamed vegetables.

variation

Baked fish in yoghurt and chive sauce

Place fish fillets in a large baking dish (nonstick if preferred), or lightly grease a normal dish. Cover with sauce and bake in moderate oven 10–15 minutes.

Serves 6.

Stir 'fried' prawns with broccoli and snow peas

If this dish is not served immediately, remove the prawns as soon as they are cooked and set aside. Make up the sauce and add the prawns just before serving. Prawns reduce in size when they are overcooked.

1 kg king green prawns (deveined, but with tail left on)
1½ cups broccoli flowerettes
2 cloves garlic, finely chopped
6–8 spring onions, chopped diagonally
100 g snow peas (topped and tailed)
1 red capsicum, seeded, sliced in fine strips
½ cup white wine
juice 3 limes
1 teaspoon fresh ginger, grated
freshly ground pepper

Heat wok, brush base with little olive oil. Add garlic, ginger and prawns, toss over high heat until prawns are just starting to turn pink. Add snow peas, spring onions and red capsicum; toss again for 1 minute. Add lime juice, white wine and freshly ground pepper. Toss for a further 2 minutes and serve immediately with rice or noodles.

Serves 4–6.

Pastry

A pastry is considered good, when it is light, tender and not too moist. However, some of the following pastries will be a little firmer with smaller amounts of fat or oil and the addition of wholemeal four. Shortcrust pastry is usually made by adding the flour and the fat, slowly pouring in enough liquid to produce a firm but light dough.

Some tips and hints for better pastry:

- start with cool ingredients
- tough pastry will result if the dough is over handled

Pizza pastry base

1½ cups wholemeal self raising flour
1 teaspoon olive oil
½ cup water
pinch cayenne pepper
extra wholemeal self raising flour to roll out the pastry

Mix all the ingredients. Add a little extra water if the pastry dough is too dry. Turn out on to a floured board and gently knead. Roll out or press the pastry into a medium sized pizza tray from edge to edge.

Makes 1 pizza base.

Sweet pastry

1 cup unbleached white flour
½ cup wholemeal self raising flour
2 tablespoons evaporated skim milk
2 tablespoons apple juice concentrate

Make the pastry by mixing the flours in a bowl then adding the skim milk and juice. Mix to a firm, hard, dough. Wrap and refrigerate at least 30–40 minutes before using.

variation

Wholemeal pastry

Recipe as sweet pastry. Omit the apple juice concentrate then add 1 tablespoon soy sauce, low salt.

Makes 1 pastry base.

Pizza 'sour' dough

1 tablespoon active dry yeast
pinch sugar *or* ¼ teaspoon apple juice concentrate
¼ cup warm water
4 cups unbleached white flour
1 cup warm water
2 tablespoons nonfat natural yoghurt
dash herb salt

Place yeast, apple juice concentrate or sugar in the ¼ cup of warm water; leave until it becomes bubbly. Add to flour and salt then mix in 1 cup warm water and yoghurt. Knead, or use a food processor. Process until dough is smooth and elastic; you may want to add more flour (only if required). Place dough in a large lightly greased bowl, cover with a tea towel and leave to rise for approximately 45 minutes. When dough has risen, break into 4 parts, roll into 4 balls, cover and leave for about 10 minutes. Roll dough into circles to cover medium size pizza plate 25 cm × 30 cm. Leave for about 10 minutes and roll a little thinner.

Makes 1 pastry base.

‘Sour’ dough pastry

1 cup unbleached white plain flour
½ cup stoneground wholemeal flour
3 tablespoons unsweetened evaporated skim milk
3 tablespoons skim milk yoghurt

Mix flours in a bowl, add the skim milk and yoghurt to make a soft but pliable dough. If mixture is too dry, add a little extra water. Roll out in the usual manner.

Makes 1 pastry base.

Sweet flan pastry

1 cup unbleached white flour
½ cup wholemeal stoneground self raising flour
2 tablespoons evaporated skim milk
½ tablespoon olive oil
⅓ cup, plus 1 tablespoon unsweetened apple juice

Mix flours in a medium bowl, add liquids and stir to make a pliable dough. Wrap in cling wrap and refrigerate for 30 minutes before using.

Makes 1 flan base.

Use nonstick pans and cake tins to eliminate the need to grease the surface with fat or oil.

Dressings, sauces, custards and dips

Dressings and sauces to enhance salads may be made from fruits, juices and vinegars and can be simple or thick mayonnaises. Fruit sauces may also be served with desserts. There are many varieties of vinegar from which to choose and, with the addition of herbs and spices, a superb recipe can be produced. Skim milk, buttermilk and nonfat yoghurts can be used together with lemons and limes. Let your imagination create different textures and flavours. Encourage the family to eat more vegetables, salads and fruits with less sugar. In this section, there is a low fat custard, and several appetising dips to be enjoyed, using avocado, chick-peas and eggplant.

Avocado and yoghurt dip

½ cup nonfat yoghurt
½ ripe avocado, peeled and cut into pieces
juice ½ lemon *or* lime (*or* 1 small lemon *or* lime)
½ teaspoon curry powder
1 spring onion, chopped
freshly ground pepper

Purée all ingredients in a blender.

Makes about 1 cup.

Azuki bolognaise sauce (no meat)

3 cups azuki beans (small type of kidney bean), soaked overnight and drained
4–6 cups water
3 onions, peeled and chopped
2 cloves garlic, finely chopped
4 cloves, whole
2 bayleaves
1 cup tomato paste
freshly ground pepper
½ cup red wine
1 carrot, peeled and finely chopped
1 celery stalk, chopped

Brush a large saucepan with light olive oil and heat. Add onion and garlic and cook gently until brown. Add celery, carrot, cloves, bayleaves and tomato paste. Stir well, cook 1 minute. Add azuki beans, 4 cups of water and the red wine, heat until boiling, stirring well. Cook for approximately 30–40 minutes, until beans are cooked, stirring occasionally, making sure sauce does not stick to base of saucepan. During cooking you may need to use extra water if sauce becomes too dry. It should be thick, about the same consistency as a good bolognaise. Season with ground pepper and use over pasta, noodles, rice etc.

Makes about 4–5 cups.

To prepare beans and lentils
Soak the beans *or* lentils in a large container of water for several hours or preferably overnight. Drain and use fresh water to cook them, unless otherwise stated.

Baba Ganoush (eggplant dip)

1 medium size eggplant
3 tablespoons tahini (sesame seed paste)
1 large clove garlic, chopped
2 tablespoons parsley, chopped
juice 1 lemon
dash herb salt

Peel eggplant, cut in half and salt heavily. Leave for 20 minutes. Rinse under cold running water, squeezing excess moisture from egg plant. Cook eggplant in a steamer or microwave until tender and soft. Cut into small pieces and purée in blender. Slowly add tahini and lemon juice and reblend. Add garlic, chopped parsley and dash herb salt. Depending on taste and thickness, a little more lemon juice can be added.

Makes about 1½–2 cups.

Banana ricotta cream

Use this on desserts and puddings in place of conventional cream:

1 cup fresh ricotta cheese, low fat
2 tablespoons evaporated skim milk
1 small ripe banana
1 tablespoon nonfat yoghurt
2 drops vanilla essence

Purée all the ingredients in a blender.

Makes about 1½ cups.

Chive dressing

1 tablespoon light olive oil
1 tablespoon chives, chopped
1 teaspoon Dijon mustard
juice of 2 small *or* 1 large lime
freshly ground pepper

Mix all the ingredients.

Makes about ½ cup.

Citrus dressing

1 tablespoon light olive oil
2 tablespoons grapefruit *or* lemon juice
dash herb salt
freshly ground pepper

Combine all the ingredients.

Makes about 3 tablespoons.

Fresh raspberry sauce

1 punnet fresh raspberries
1 teaspoon brown sugar
1 tablespoon fresh orange juice

Purée all the ingredients in a blender.

variations

Fresh strawberry sauce

Recipe as above. Omit the raspberries and use 1 punnet of fresh strawberries, washed and hulled.

Fresh blackberry sauce

Recipe as above. Omit the raspberries and add 1 punnet of fresh blackberries.

Makes about 1 cup.

Fresh tomato sauce

500 g ripe tomatoes *or* 1 large can tomatoes, low salt
1 clove garlic, finely chopped
1 small onion, finely chopped
1 teaspoon tomato paste
1 teaspoon basil
1 sprig thyme
¼ teaspoon oregano
freshly ground pepper

Remove the skins from the fresh tomatoes (if used). Do this by pouring boiling water over them. Peel and chop. If using canned tomatoes, drain, cut in half, and if preferred, remove the seeds by squeezing. Gently sauté the onion and garlic in a nonstick pan or a pan lightly brushed with olive oil. Add chopped tomatoes, thyme and tomato paste, simmer for 10–15 minutes. Add oregano, basil and freshly ground pepper, cook for a further 2 minutes and use as required.

Makes about 1½–2 cups.

Fruit glaze

1 sachet gelatine, dissolved in hot water

Dissolve the gelatine in the water and cool. Carefully brush over the fruit as directed. You may use agar agar *or* aspic in place of the gelatine.

variation

Coloured fruit glaze

Recipe as above. Add a few drops of pink, red or green colouring to the glaze. If you wish a natural colour, use beetroot juice for red and parsley juice for green.

'Green' lime and ricotta sauce

2 tablespoons fresh ricotta cheese, low fat
1 tablespoon nonfat yoghurt
1 tablespoon fresh parsley, chopped
1 teaspoon fresh chives, chopped
1 teaspoon fresh lime juice
pinch basil or dill

Purée all the ingredients in a blender and use at once.

Makes about ¼ cup.

Herbed French dressing

1 tablespoon light olive oil
1 tablespoon cider vinegar
1 dessertspoon tamari *or* soy sauce, low salt
1 large clove garlic, chopped
1 dessertspoon parsley, chopped
1 spring onion, chopped

Combine all the ingredients and refrigerate. Stir before serving.

Makes about ¼ cup.

Hommas (chick-pea dip)

150 g chick-peas (soaked overnight in 4 cups water)
1 clove garlic
1 tablespoon fresh parsley
juice 1 large lemon
1–2 tablespoons tahini
dash herb salt
freshly ground pepper

Cook chick-peas in the overnight soaking water for approximately 2–3 hours until tender — add more water if necessary. Set aside to cool. Chop garlic and parsley in blender or food processor; add cooled, drained, chick-peas, tahini and lemon juice. Add herb salt and freshly ground pepper.

Lime and yoghurt dressing

½ cup nonfat yoghurt
1 large clove garlic, finely chopped
juice of 1 lime
dash herb salt
freshly ground pepper

Combine all the ingredients.

Makes about ½ cup.

Store salad dressings, low in fat in the refrigerator and use as required. You may need to add a little skim milk if the recipe has thickened.

Orange ricotta sauce

Delicious with desserts.

1½ cups fresh nonfat ricotta cheese
juice of 1 large, sweet, orange

Purée all the ingredients in a blender.

Makes about 1½ cups.

variation

Vanilla ricotta sauce

Recipe as above. Omit the orange juice, add ½ cup skim milk and ½ teaspoon vanilla essence.

Raspberry sauce (cooked)

1 punnet of fresh *or* frozen raspberries
½ cup apple juice concentrate
1 tablespoon arrowroot
dash of Kirsch (optional)

Place the raspberries in a small saucepan and simmer very slowly until cooked, about 10 minutes. Add the remaining ingredients. Stir as the sauce thickens. Cool, or serve hot over fruits or desserts of choice.

Makes about 1 cup.

Skim milk vanilla custard 1

1½ cups water
¼ cup skim milk powder
2 tablespoons apple juice concentrate
2 tablespoons cornflour
½ tablespoon vanilla essence
1 banana, peeled and puréed
1 tablespoon brandy (optional)
freshly grated nutmeg

Combine water, skim milk powder, apple juice concentrate and brandy in a small saucepan. Mix cornflour with a little water to make a paste and gradually add to the mixture. Slowly heat and gently stir until the mixture has thickened. Add the puréed banana, mixed with a little of the custard, stir well. Add the grated nutmeg and vanilla essence.

Makes about 1½ cups.

Skim milk custard 2

1½ cups water
¼ cup skim milk powder
2 tablespoons apple juice concentrate
½ teaspoon vanilla essence
2 tablespoons cornflour
1 banana, puréed
1 tablespoon brandy (optional)
1 sachet gelatine* dissolved in a little hot water
freshly grated nutmeg

Combine the water, skim milk powder, apple juice concentrate and brandy in a small saucepan. Gently mix the cornflour with a little water and stir into the mixture. Slowly heat and gently stir as the mixture thickens. Add the puréed banana, vanilla essence and the nutmeg. Allow to cool and carefully fold in the dissolved gelatine.

Makes about 1½ cups.

* You can substitute the gelatine with agar agar *or* aspic and use in the same manner.

Skim milk white sauce

1 tablespoon unbleached white flour
½ cup evaporated skim milk
1½ cups skim milk
¼ teaspoon nutmeg
little black pepper

Mix flour to a paste with a little milk, add remaining milk and slowly cook until sauce thickens. Add nutmeg.

Sauces using basic skim milk white sauce

Anchovy sauce

Use over poached *or* boiled fish.
Make up the sauce and add anchovy essence to taste.

Egg sauce

Use over poached *or* boiled fish.
Make up the sauce and add 2 hard boiled eggs *or* egg whites cut into strips.

Cheese sauce

Use over fish *or* vegetables.
Make up the sauce and add 60 g grated cheese, low fat. Mix well into the sauce as it cooks.

Onion sauce

Use over roast lamb.

Make up the sauce and add 1 small onion, diced, when the sauce is cooking. You can also add chopped parsley to this recipe.

Mushroom sauce

Use with omelette.

Make up the sauce and add 4 button mushrooms, chopped, and 2 tablespoons parsley, chopped.

Mustard sauce

Serve over grilled fish.

Make up the sauce and add diluted English mustard for a fairly hot sauce.

Parsley sauce

Serve over poached *or* boiled fish *or* vegetables.

Make up the sauce and add 1 teaspoon parsley, chopped.

Soy and yoghurt dressing

¼ cup spring onions, chopped
¼ cup parsley, chopped
¼ cup fresh coriander, chopped
2 tablespoons tamari *or* soy sauce, low salt
1 tablespoon fresh ginger, grated
3 tablespoons nonfat yoghurt
2 tablespoons cider vinegar

Combine all the ingredients and refrigerate.

Makes about 1 cup.

Tahini and yoghurt sauce

1 cup nonfat yoghurt
3 tablespoons tahini
1 clove garlic
juice ½ lemon
½ teaspoon dill
1 tablespoon fresh parsley, chopped

Purée all the ingredients in a blender and serve.

Makes about 1¼ cups.

Tamari and honey dressing

1 tablespoon olive oil
1 dessertspoon tamari *or* soy sauce, low salt
1 tablespoon fresh lemon *or* lime juice
1 teaspoon honey

Combine all the ingredients.

Makes about ¼ cup.

Tarragon and yoghurt dressing

½ cup nonfat yoghurt
1 tablespoon cider vinegar
1 teaspoon tarragon
1 teaspoon Dijon mustard
dash herb salt
freshly ground pepper

Mix all the ingredients and refrigerate before serving.

Makes about ½ cup.

White sauce (thick)

2 tablespoons unbleached white flour
1 cup of low fat *or* skim milk
1 tablespoon evaporated skim milk
1 teaspoon lemon juice
pinch nutmeg
pinch cayenne pepper
pinch freshly ground pepper

Mix flour to a paste with a little skim milk and slowly add remaining liquid. Place in a saucepan over gentle heat and bring to the boil, stirring constantly until sauce is thick. Add nutmeg, cayenne and pepper.

For a thinner white sauce you require:
1 tablespoon unbleached white flour
1¼ cups skim milk, the remaining ingredients, and method, as above.

Roasting vegetables
All vegetables including potatoes, pumpkin, parsnips, carrots, sweet potato (white or orange), can be dry roasted and served with a roast meal. It is often a good idea to steam them lightly first, and then pop them in the oven on the tray to roast. They may be wrapped in foil or in a glad bag — this will allow them to cook quicker. However, to brown the vegetables, open the foil or bag about 20 minutes before completion time.

Casseroles may be thickened with cornflour and/or arrowroot. Add extra fibre by using rolled oats or wholegrain flours.

Eat dried fruits e.g. apricots, dates, sultanas (raisins), apple, banana, pineapple or commercial fruit leathers.

Sugar

Recipes to help you reduce your sugar intake.

When preparing food:

- use less sugar in home prepared foods such as cakes and biscuits
- use fruit juices in cooking and sautés
- make cakes without sugar
- make desserts with natural fruit as a sweetener
- use spices such as cinnamon, nutmeg, ginger and allspice to enhance the flavour of the foods

Cakes and desserts

Most people have a sweet tooth that demands to be satisfied every now and then. What better way to satisfy your craving than to use these recipes? They will be difficult to resist. Many of these delectable recipes are actually cooked without added sugar, and have little or no added fats. Yet — they are tasty and very moreish! Fruits, dried fruits and natural juice sweeteners are used to sweeten and flavour the recipes.

Oatbran, as widely publicised, is found to lower blood cholesterol levels and is also rich in soluble fibre.

Oatbran muffins are a great way to eat oatbran and, used regularly, a nonstick 12-cup muffin tray would be a good investment.

Apple raisin meringue pie

A quantity of sweet pastry, recipe page 68.

filling
2 cups cooked apples
¼ cup water
¼ cup orange juice
1 cup raisins
2–3 teaspoons orange rind, grated, (minus pith)
sprinkle ground cloves
¼ teaspoon cinnamon

meringue
2 egg whites
2 tablespoons evaporated skim milk

Preheat oven to 200°C. Prepare filling by placing raisins, orange juice, rind and water in small saucepan and simmer for approximately 10–15 minutes. Cool. When cooled, mix with apples, cloves and cinnamon. Roll out pastry and line a flan tin. Spoon apple filling into pastry. Make topping by beating egg whites until stiff and gently fold in evaporated skim milk. Spread meringue on top of apples. Bake for 15–20 minutes until pastry is cooked and meringue perfectly golden.

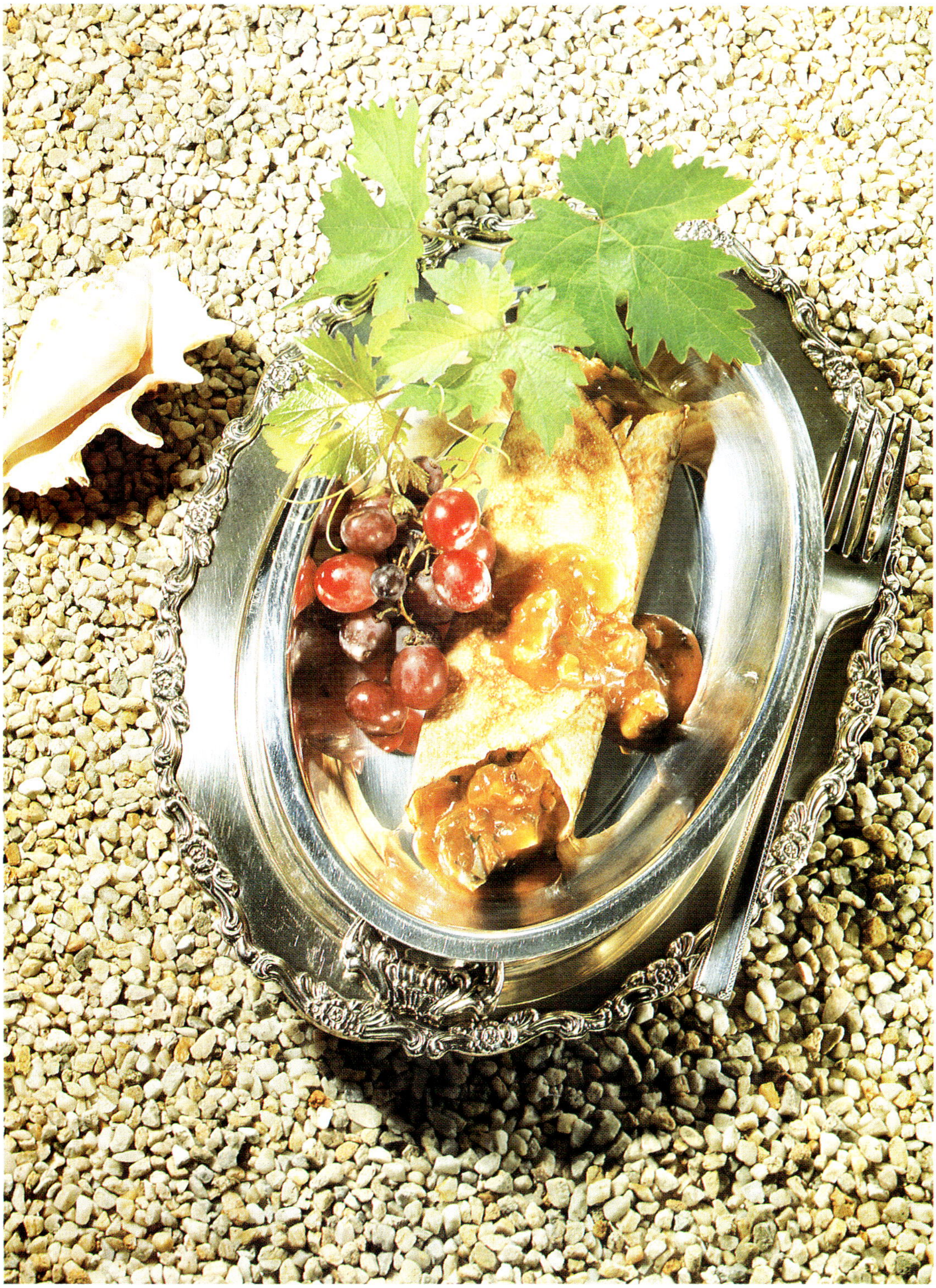

Seafood crêpes (*page 65*)

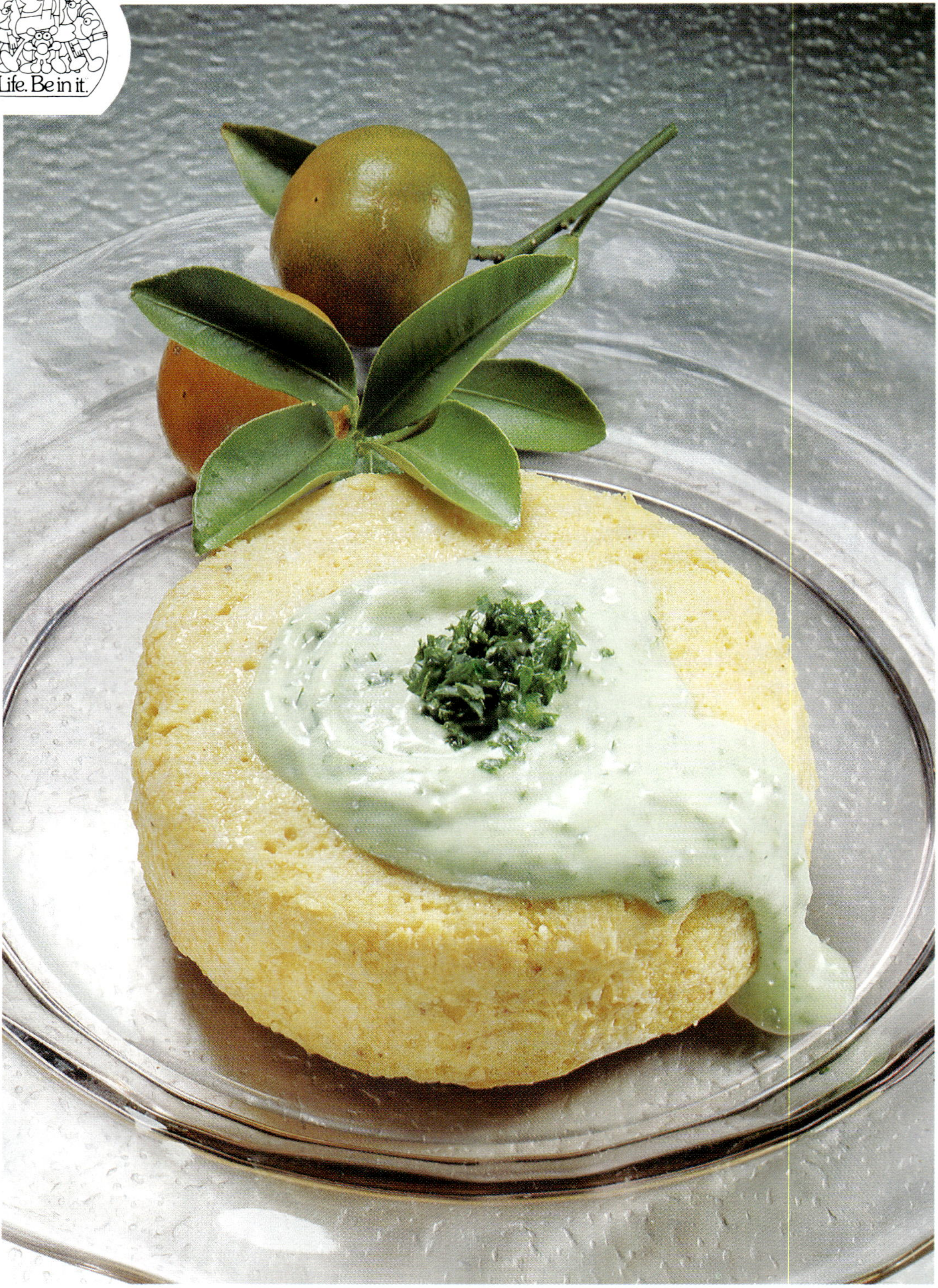

Pumpkin timbales (*page 117*)
'Green' lime and ricotta sauce (*page 76*)

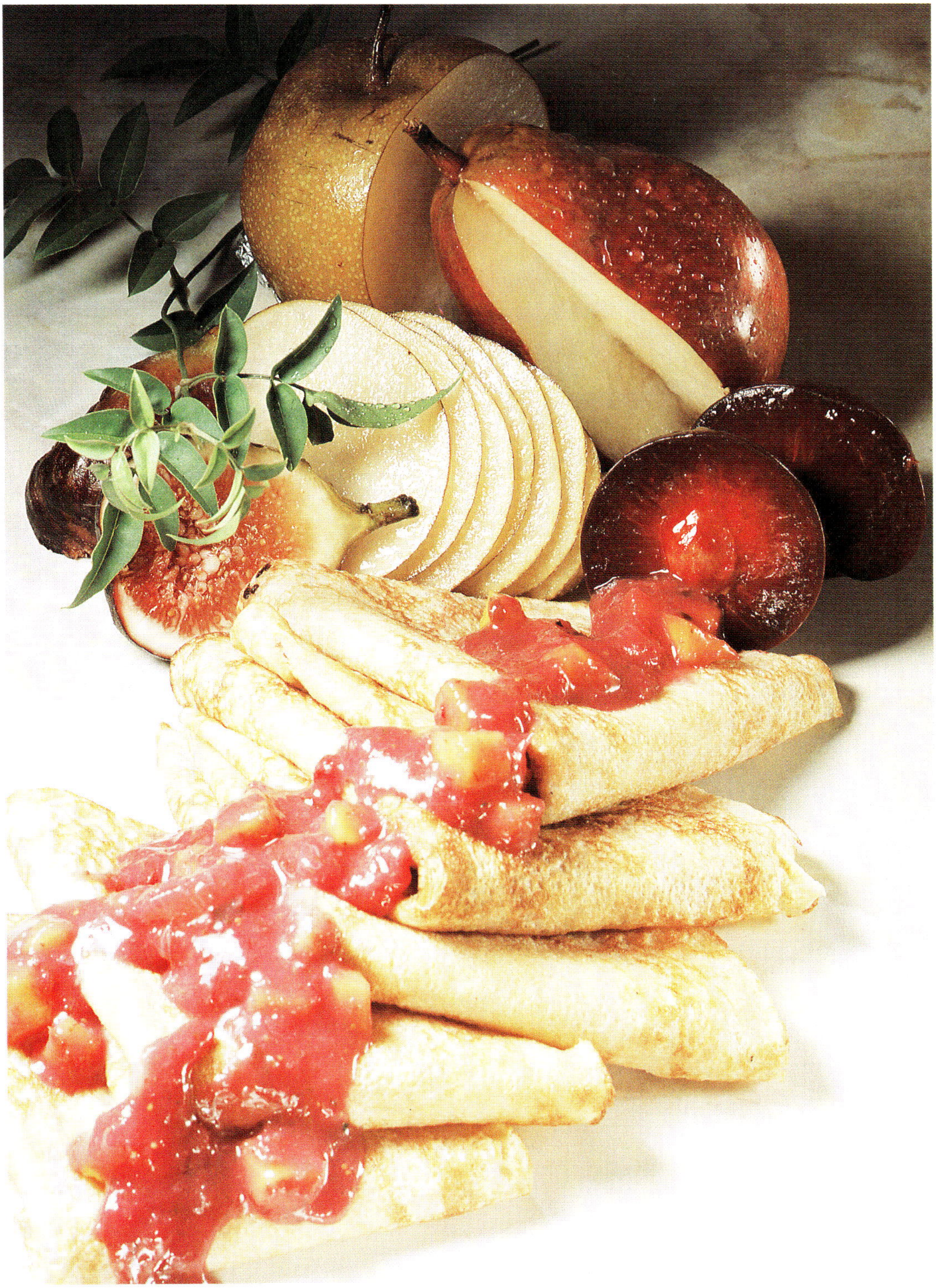

Blintzes (*page 136*)
Mango, plum and fig dessert (*page 138*)

Life. Be in it.

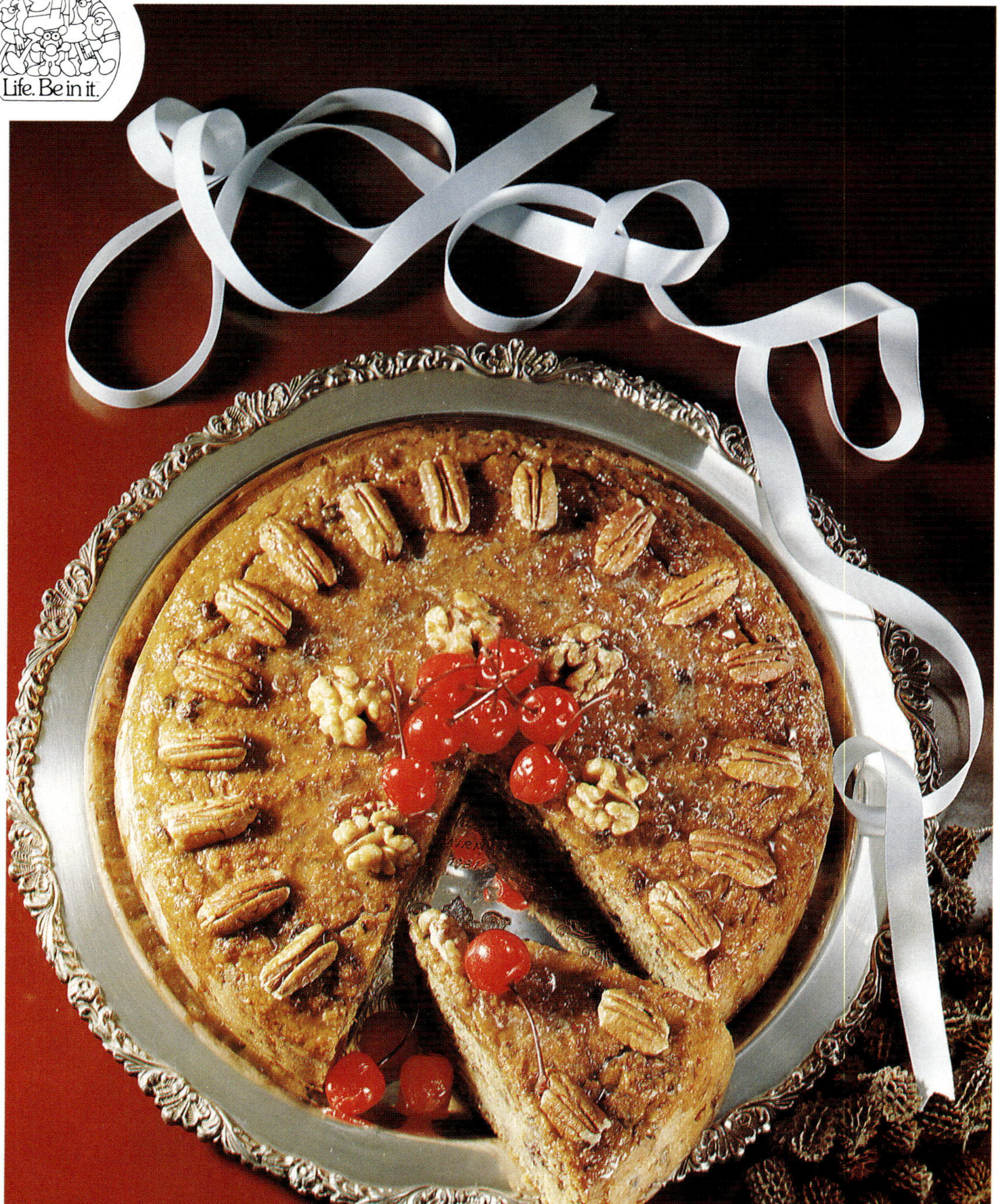

Pumpkin fruit cake (*page 90*)

variation

Apple and apricot meringue

Recipe as above. Use 1½ cups apple and ½ cup dried apricots soaked in ½ cup water.

Banana and apricot oat muffins

1 cup oatbran
¾ cup wholemeal self raising flour
¼ cup wheatgerm
½ cup fresh orange juice
½ cup dried apricots, chopped
1 ripe banana
½ cup skim milk
2 tablespoons evaporated skim milk
2 egg whites
1 tablespoon light oil

Preheat oven to 220°C. Place orange juice and dried apricots in a small saucepan, bring to boil, stir, and set aside to cool. Combine oatbran, flour and wheatgerm; add skim milk, eggs and mix. Finally, add mashed banana, orange juice and apricots. Mix thoroughly, fill muffin tray and bake for 15 minutes or until golden brown.

Makes 12 muffins or 7–8 large muffins.

Mixed fruit flan

1 quantity of sweet flan pastry, recipe page 70
1 quantity of skim milk custard, recipe page 79
1 425 g can peaches in natural juice, drained
1 425 g can apricots in natural juice, drained
1 punnet large strawberries, washed, hulled and halved
2 kiwi fruit, peeled and sliced longways

topping
1 quantity of fruit glaze, recipe page 76

Line a large flan base with the pastry and bake blind according to instructions. Pour in the prepared custard and allow to set. Arrange the fruit on to the set custard, taking care to decorate carefully with the fruit in an alternating pattern to cover the top. Gently brush the glaze over the fruit and allow to set.

variations

Strawberry fruit flan

Recipe as above. Omit the mixed fruit and decorate with 1½–2 punnets of strawberries, hulled and halved.

Pineapple fruit flan

Recipe as above. Omit the mixed fruit and decorate with unsweetened pineapple pieces drained, or rings of unsweetened pineapple. Place a glacé cherry in the centre of each pineapple ring before brushing with the glaze.

Cherry fruit flan

Recipe as above. Omit the mixed fruit and decorate with 2 cans of black cherries, drained. Glaze as directed.

Orange oatbran muffins

1 cup oatbran
½ cup wholemeal self raising flour
½ cup wheatgerm
1 tablespoon apple juice concentrate
2 egg whites
2 tablespoons evaporated skim milk
2 tablespoons sultanas
1 tablespoon light oil
½ cup fresh orange juice
¼ cup skim milk
2 tablespoons orange rind, grated

Preheat oven to 220°C. Mix oatbran, flour, wheatgerm and orange peel. Add eggs, skim milk, orange juice, apple juice concentrate, oil and sultanas. Mix thoroughly. Fill muffin tray and bake 15 minutes or until muffins are golden brown.

Makes 12 medium size muffins or 2–8 large muffins.

Oatbran muffins

2 cups oatbran
1 tablespoon apple juice concentrate
½ cup rolled oats
¼ cup walnuts, chopped
¼ cup sultanas
¾ cup skim milk
2 tablespoons evaporated skim milk
2 egg whites
1 tablespoon light olive oil
1 tablespoon baking powder

topping
extra rolled oats

Preheat oven to 220°C. Combine oatbran with baking powder, add walnuts, sultanas and mix through. Add rolled oats, skim milk, eggs, oil, apple juice concentrate and mix thoroughly. Fill muffin tray with mix, top with some rolled oats, and bake approximately 15 minutes or until golden brown.

Makes 12 small-to-medium size muffins or 7–8 large muffins.

Pumpkin fruit cake

This fruit cake may be made up and served as a Christmas cake during the Festive Season.

500 g butternut pumpkin, peeled and chopped
2 cups unsweetened apple juice
500 g mixed dried fruit, e.g., dates, sultanas, raisins, currants
500 g stoneground wholemeal flour
2 teaspoons baking powder
6 egg whites, lightly whisked
¼ teaspoon ground cloves
½ teaspoon mixed spice, e.g., cinnamon, ginger, nutmeg
2 cups unsweetened apple juice (extra)

decoration
½ cup almonds *or* pecan nuts and glacé cherries

Preheat oven to 150°C. Place the pumpkin and apple juice in a saucepan and gently simmer until soft. Drain and mash (reserve the juice). Place the dried fruit and apple juice into another saucepan and boil, then simmer for 15 minutes; set aside and cool in the juice. Place the cooked fruit in a large bowl, add the spices, mashed pumpkin and slowly stir in the flour. Mix well, adding the egg whites and the left-over juice from the pumpkin. The mixture should be quite wet. Pour into a lined cake tin. Decorate with the nuts of choice and bake 2–2½ hours. Test with a skewer in the centre to see if the cake is cooked. When cooked, leave in the tin for approximately 10 minutes.

Grains and cereals

Recipes to help you eat more grains and cereals:

- for a healthy diet, eat at least four servings of bread *or* other cereal each day
- 1 serving is approximately 1 slice of bread *or* 1 cup of ready-to-serve cereal, pasta or rice
- these provide fibre from the B group of vitamins

Add extra flavour to the following:
Pasta: cardamon, coriander, garlic, mace, marjoram, mint and oregano
Rice: curry, mace, marjoram, paprika, saffron, sage and thyme

The fibre content of food is not affected by any cooking process. However, when foods containing fibre are sieved, valuable fibre should not be discarded, that is, the material left behind. If it is not to be used in the recipe, place into your soup.

Breads, scones, crêpes and cereals

Bread has always been considered the *staff of life*.

Now, with the nutritional emphasis on adding more complex carbohydrates and fibre into our diet, many new varieties of wholegrain bread have been introduced.

These include grains not previously considered, e.g., rye, oats, triticale and barley, which are now frequently used.

New combinations of cereal grains allow the consumer greater choice, and the addition of oatbran to our diet is a sound idea to assist us to lower and maintain our levels of cholesterol.

Beer bread

2 cups unbleached white flour
1 cup stoneground wholemeal self raising flour
2 teaspoons baking powder
1 dessertspoon brown sugar *or* 2 teaspoons apple juice concentrate
1 can beer

Preheat oven to 180°C. Mix all ingredients. Line a loaf tin with baking paper, or use a nonstick loaf tin. Place bread dough in tin and cook for 45–50 minutes or until golden in colour.

Add more fibre to your diet by introducing wholegrain breads, 'sour' dough, pita breads and rice cakes. For nutritious lunches, fill slices or pockets in the breads with a variety of salad vegetables.

Buttermilk herb bread

¼ cup warm water
1 tablespoon active dry yeast
2 teaspoons apple juice concentrate
3 cups unbleached white flour
2 egg whites
¼ teaspoon thyme
¼ teaspoon marjoram
¼ teaspoon oregano
1 tablespoon light oil
¾ cup buttermilk

Preheat oven to 200°C. Dissolve yeast with apple juice concentrate in warm water in a large bowl or food processor bowl. Leave until it becomes bubbly. Mix herbs with flour and add to yeast-and-water mix. Warm buttermilk (not hot, just warm), and add to flour mixture. Combine. Add oil and egg, mix through. If making by hand, knead dough for about 10 minutes or use processor for about 12–15 seconds until dough is stiff but firm and elastic. Put dough in a large bowl, cover with towel and let rise in a warm place for about 1 hour. Shape into loaf and place in a nonstick loaf tin (or lightly greased loaf tin). Cover again, let rise for another 35–45 minutes. Bake approximately 35–40 minutes or until it is golden brown.

Herb and pumpkin damper

3 cups stoneground wholemeal self raising flour
¾ cup skim milk
¼ cup evaporated skim milk
1 cup cooked pumpkin, mashed (dash nutmeg)
2 tablespoon parsley, chopped
½ teaspoon marjoram
1 tablespoon nonfat yoghurt

Preheat oven to 240°C. Mix flour, marjoram and parsley in a bowl, make a well in centre and add milk. Mix through. Add pumpkin and yoghurt, mix well and turn on to floured board. Knead mixture until fairly smooth and shape into a round. Place on a baking tray brushed with milk or a touch of light oil or, cook on a nonstick floured tray and brush with a little milk. Bake in hot oven, 240°C for 15 minutes, then reduce heat to 210°C and bake for a further 15 minutes until risen and golden brown.

Wholemeal cheese scones

3 cups stoneground wholemeal self raising flour
½ cup grated cheese, low fat
¾ cup water *or* skim milk
generous pinch cayenne pepper
extra wholemeal self raising flour to roll out the dough

topping
¼ cup grated cheese, low fat
1 tablespoon nonfat yoghurt

Preheat the oven to 200°C. Mix all the ingredients to make a scone dough, adding a little extra water if the mixture is too dry. Turn the dough on to a well floured board. Gently knead the dough and roll out into a large scone. Cut into rounds with a scone cutter. Brush with the yoghurt and top with the grated cheese. Place the scones on to a floured tray and bake about 15 minutes or until cooked.

variation

Sweet wholemeal scones

Recipe as above. Omit cayenne pepper. Add ½ cup dates, chopped and pitted.

Wholemeal herb and onion scones

Recipe and instructions as for wholemeal cheese scones. Add 1 small onion, finely chopped, sautéd and cooled, and a generous pinch of herbs of your choice.

Makes about 12 scones.

As butter and oil have been omitted in this recipe, a sprinkle of water on each scone is required before reheating in the oven or microwave — later on, or the next day. They make delightful low cal/kJ crunchy scones.

Wholemeal crêpes

½ cup stoneground wholemeal plain flour
½ cup unbleached white flour
1–1½ cups skim milk
1 egg*

Mix the flours in a medium bowl, make a well in the centre, add the egg and stir until egg is absorbed. Slowly add the milk, making sure the mixture is of a smooth consistency. It should be fairly thin. Beat well and set aside for an hour. To make the crêpes, use a nonstick pan or a pan lightly brushed with olive oil. Heat until hot, add a spoonful of the mixture — enough to spread over the base of the pan. When golden on the under side, turn over and lightly cook the other side. Always keep the pan hot for each crêpe.

* You may use the white only, if preferred.

variation

Buckwheat crêpes

Recipe as above. Use only ¼ cup unbleached white flour and ¼ cup buckwheat flour.

Makes about 6 crêpes.

Yorkshire pudding

1 cup unbleached white flour
2 cups skim milk
1 egg white, plus 1 whole egg
little olive oil

Sieve flour into a basin and make a well in the centre. Break in the egg white plus the whole egg, add half the liquid and whisk to a smooth mixture, gradually adding the rest of the liquid and then allowing to rest. Select a shallow pan, 12 cm in diameter. Brush pan with a little light olive oil, pour in batter and cook in hot oven for approximately 15 minutes.

Serves 4–6.

Pasta, rice and beans

Wholegrain pastas are now available in many varieties for cooking. They make superb salads, spaghetti, and help thicken vegetable soups. With the addition of beans and lentils into the diet, protein intake will be assured. Home made baked beans on toast is a nutritional and sustaining meal — use for light lunches and easy suppers. It is great for the little ones. Brown rice may take a little longer to cook; it has a nutty taste, plenty of fibre and is well worth the waiting time. Use white rice as an alternative and wild rice for variety.

Boiled rice (brown)

1½ cups brown rice
3 cups water

Wash rice well in a strainer. Place in a saucepan with water, bring to boil, lower heat and simmer, covered, for approximately 35–40 minutes until rice is just cooked and all the water has been absorbed.

You can use boiled rice as an accompaniment to curries, vegetable or meat dishes etc. It can also be refrigerated and used when required e.g., 'fried' rice, in salads or as a cereal.

variations

White rice

Recipe and instructions as above. However, white rice will cook much quicker, so only cook for 15–20 minutes.

Wild rice

This is usually a mixture of different rices and is not strictly wild. It does have a lovely flavour and also adds colour to a meal.

Recipe and instructions as per rice packet.

Curried rice

1½ cups cooked, brown rice, cold, recipe page 96
1 small brown onion
1½ teaspoon curry powder
½ teaspoon turmeric
½ teaspoon ground cumin

In a large pan, brushed with a hint of light olive oil, gently sauté onion, curry powder, turmeric and cumin, for approximately 2–3 minutes. Add rice and mix thoroughly. Serve with stir 'fry' vegetables, fish or lamb.

Serves 4.

Eastern noodle stir 'fry'

300 g thin dried wheat noodles,* in cakes
2 large onions, peeled and thinly sliced
1 clove garlic, finely chopped
2 chicken breasts, steamed (skin and fat removed)
1 cup fresh bean sprouts
1 rasher bacon, chopped (rind and fat removed)
1 teaspoon ginger, freshly grated
1–2 tablespoons tamari *or* soy sauce, low salt
1 crisp green lettuce (e.g., cos), washed and dried
handful spring onion stems, chopped

Cook noodles in boiling water for 3 minutes, gently breaking cakes apart. Drain thoroughly under cold water then set aside. Brush wok with a little light olive oil. Heat and cook onions, garlic, ginger and bacon for approximately 5 minutes, stirring repeatedly to avoid burning.

Slice cooked chicken thinly, then cut into cubes. Add to wok, toss 1 minute then gradually add noodles, tossing well to mix through. Heat until hot, add bean sprouts and soy sauce. Shred lettuce and arrange on serving platter. Pile noodle mixture on top and sprinkle with the chopped spring onions.

Serves 4.

* These noodles are available from health food stores or Asian food shops.

Life. Be in it.

Fettucine vegetable 'cream'

For additional flavour, season with herb salt and top with freshly grated parmesan cheese.

1 cup broccoli flowerettes
1 medium zucchini, sliced
2 small carrots, sliced and peeled
125 g fresh green beans, cut in half (topped and tailed)
500 g fettucine
1½ cups fresh ricotta cheese, low fat, *or* 1½ cups nonfat cottage cheese
½–1 cup skim milk
1 dessertspoon fresh basil, chopped *or* 2 teaspoons dried basil
1 tablespoon fresh chives, chopped
¼ cup fresh parsley, chopped
freshly ground pepper

Steam all vegetables until just tender. Place fettucine in boiling water until cooked, then drain. Purée ricotta or cottage cheese in blender, add skim milk, basil, chives and parsley. Return vegetables to a nonstick pan, add fettucine and combine sauce over top. Stir through and slowly heat until warm. Serve with a sprig of fresh basil and a little pepper. Serve with homemade bread or damper and a green salad.

Serves 4–6.

Vitamins
A good mixed diet will provide all the vitamins necessary to good health. They are present in small amounts in different foods and are essential to life.

‘Fried’ rice (vegetarian)

This is a very versatile dish. Serve as a main course, entrée, garnish, or a wonderful salad.

2 cups cooked, brown rice, cold, recipe page 96
2 egg whites
3 spring onions
1 carrot, peeled and finely chopped
1 celery stalk, finely diced
½ red *or* green pepper
1 tablespoon tamari *or* soy sauce, low salt
handful fresh parsley, chopped

Whisk egg whites with fork and cook in nonstick pan (covering entire base of pan), until golden on one side; turn, and cook for 1 minute. Set aside on a plate.

Heat wok or large pan until hot, brushing the base with a little olive oil. Add spring onions, carrot, celery and green pepper and cook for 3 minutes, tossing vegetables once or twice making sure they do not burn. Add rice and mix thoroughly. Stir in soy sauce. Slice egg into thin strips, cut in half and sprinkle over rice with the chopped fresh parsley.

variations

‘Fried’ rice with chicken

Recipe as above, *add*
1 cup chicken, diced (skinned)

‘Fried’ rice with prawns and shrimps

Recipe as above, *add*
¼ kg fresh prawns, cooked
¼ kg fresh shrimps

Serves 4.

Green fettucine with fresh tomato sauce

400 g green fettucine

1 quantity fresh tomato sauce, recipe page 75
cheese, freshly grated, low fat *or* Italian parmesan, freshly grated

Prepare tomato sauce as per recipe. Cook fettucine in boiling water, according to directions on packet — less time if fettucine is fresh, not dried. When just tender, drain and serve with fresh tomato sauce and sprinkle with either of above cheeses.

variation

Fettucine Italienne

If you have the time, eggplant tastes much better when char-grilled on a barbecue.

Recipe as above, *add*
1 small eggplant, peeled and cut into cubes
1 cup button mushrooms, sliced

Either steam eggplant and mushrooms and add to sauce or gently sauté in a small pan lightly brushed with olive oil.

Serves 4.

Peas
Newly picked fresh peas, contain plenty of vitamin C. When cooked, they lose about half of the original amount of vitamin C.

Lentil pie

This makes a handsome centre piece, served either hot or cold.

1 quantity wholemeal pastry, recipe page 69 *or* 2–3 sheets of ready rolled wholemeal shortcrust pastry
1½ cups brown lentils, washed and drained
1 large brown onion, finely chopped
2 cloves garlic, minced *or* finely chopped
5 egg whites
2 cups skim milk
½ cup fresh parsley, chopped
1 tablespoon curry powder
¼ teaspoon nutmeg
½ teaspoon coriander
freshly ground pepper

Cook lentils in 4–5 cups of water. Bring to boil and simmer for about 20–30 minutes until cooked. Add extra water if necessary, but almost all the liquid should have evaporated. Drain and set aside. Roll out pastry and line base and sides of a 20 cm × 8 cm nonstick baking tin (if nonstick is not available, brush sparingly with light olive oil). Heat a pan, brush with minimum light olive oil and gently cook garlic, onion and curry powder, to extract the most flavour. Add nutmeg, coriander and freshly ground pepper. Toss through. Add drained lentils and mix all ingredients thoroughly. Whisk egg whites lightly with fork, add skim milk and parsley. Place lentil mixture in pastry and pour egg and milk over top of lentils making sure it seeps through by using a fork to loosen lentil mixture. Cover top of pie with remaining pastry, decorate with pastry leaves and cook in a moderate oven for approximately 60–70 minutes or until done. Test with a skewer.

Pasta salad with beans and pinenuts

For a colourful presentation, toast *half* the pinenuts until golden brown, then mix with the untoasted pinenuts.

250 g wholemeal pasta, medium size e.g., shells
250 g button mushrooms, finely sliced
250 g fresh green beans (topped and tailed)
1 tablespoon fresh chives, chopped
2 tablespoons pinenuts, toasted
Citrus dressing, recipe page 74

Cook wholemeal pasta in boiling water until just cooked. *Do not overcook*. Drain and rinse well. Cut beans into approximately 5 cm pieces and blanch in boiling water for 5 minutes or microwave until just tender. Drain and refresh under cold water. Arrange pasta and beans in serving bowl and sprinkle with sliced mushrooms and chives. Mix dressing, and when ready to serve, pour over and sprinkle with toasted pinenuts.

Serves 4.

Rice salad

1½ cups brown rice cooked in 3 cups water until cooked, and all water is absorbed. (It is preferable that rice is cooked the day before, giving a better result to the salad.)
3 spring onions, finely chopped
1 celery stalk, finely diced
2 tablespoons parsley, chopped
2 tablespoons pinenuts, toasted

Place rice, onions, parsley and pinenuts in a bowl. In a small jar or bowl mix 1 tablespoon olive oil, juice of half a grapefruit, 1 clove garlic (finely chopped), and a little ground pepper. Pour over rice salad and serve.

Serves 4–6.

Pasta with mussels and broccoli

For added presentation, leave a few mussels in their shells and add one to each serve.

500 g wholemeal thin spaghetti
2 kg fresh mussels (cleaned)
2 cups broccoli flowerettes
1 cup white wine and 1 cup of fish stock, recipe page 26 (for cooking mussels), *or* 1½ cups fresh stock, recipe page 24, and ½ cup cider vinegar
2 cloves garlic, chopped *or* finely minced
1 pinch saffron (available from chemist *or* speciality delicatessen)
liquid from cooked mussels
2 tablespoons nonfat yoghurt
freshly ground pepper

In a large saucepan heat white wine, or stock and vinegar, and cook mussels (about 6 at a time), by simmering until they open. Remove with slotted spoon to bowl and take mussels from their shells and set aside. When all mussels are cooked, discard cooking liquid, retaining any liquid in bowl from opened mussels. Cook broccoli in boiling water for 3–4 minutes, drain and set aside. Cook spaghetti in boiling water until cooked. While pasta is cooking, brush a large saucepan with a little light olive oil and gently sauté garlic. Add reserved liquid from opened mussels, add saffron, heat through, gently. Stir in yoghurt. Drain pasta, return to sauce and toss through. Add the mussels and broccoli, toss all ingredients over low heat, sprinkle with a little ground pepper and serve.

Serves 4–6.

Did you know that a single grain of wheat has three parts? The germ is the seed, there is a starchy part, and the bran or fibrous outer layer is the covering.

Spaghetti with fresh asparagus

Fresh asparagus should be tied with a string when cooking. The end of the tie should be left long, like a fishing line, making it easy to pull out of the water to test for taste.

400 g wholemeal spaghetti *or* tagliatelle
2 bunches fresh asparagus
½ cup fresh chives, chopped
1 clove garlic, finely chopped
¼ cup parsley, freshly chopped
1 tablespoon Dijon mustard
½ teaspoon thyme
2 tablespoons water (from asparagus *or* pasta cooking water)

Place asparagus in enough boiling to cover it and cook for approximately 3 minutes. *Do not overcook*. Cook pasta in boiling water as directed. While pasta is cooking, combine mustard, chives, parsley, garlic and thyme and 2 tablespoons of asparagus water or pasta water. Drain pasta, stir sauce through asparagus, sprinkle with freshly ground pepper and serve warm.

variation

Spaghetti with chicken and fresh asparagus

Recipe as above but add 2 chicken breasts, skin removed. Steam chicken breasts until tender and slice into thin strips or, if preferred, cut into small pieces.

Serves 4.

Spinach ravioli with walnuts and chives

750 g fresh spinach and ricotta ravioli*
¾ cup walnuts, cut in half
2 tablespoons yoghurt, nonfat
1 egg white
¾ cup cheese, low fat, freshly grated
½ teaspoon basil
freshly ground pepper
handful fresh chives, chopped

Cook ravioli in boiling salted water for 3–4 minutes. Drain well and return to pan. Beat egg white and half the grated cheese with a fork and add to pasta; toss through off the heat. Add yoghurt, basil, half the walnuts and half the chives. Stir gently over low heat until yoghurt is very warm. Serve in a large heated dish and sprinkle with remaining walnuts, grated cheese and chives.

Serves 4–6.

Spinach is a vegetable that is low in cal/kJ. Its leaves can be used in salads, hot vegetable dishes or eaten as a side vegetable. It has a high fibre content and contains vitamins A and C.

* Fresh spinach and ricotta ravioli are available from a good delicatessen or a speciality pasta shop.

Tabouli

1 cup bourghul (cracked wheat)
2 cups boiling water
2 tomatoes, chopped
1 small onion, chopped
½ cup parsley, chopped
1 dessertspoon fresh mint, chopped
juice 1 lemon
1 tablespoon light olive oil
freshly ground pepper

Soak bourghul in boiling water for 1 hour until all water is absorbed. Squeeze out excess.

Combine bourghul with all remaining ingredients and refrigerate until ready to serve.

Serves 4.

By eating more high fibre vegetables, fruits and wholegrains, there is less risk of developing many of the illnesses ranging from obesity to cancer.

Vegetables

Recipes to help you eat more vegetables:

- choose fresh vegetables in season, when there is more variety, better quality, and prices are lower
- vegetables are low in fat and food energy and high in vitamins and minerals
- vegetables provide a variety of tastes, textures and colours to meals and are easy to prepare

For a healthy diet, include in meals selection at least once per day:

- one serving (about ½ a cup), of a leafy green or orange vegetable for vitamin A
- one serving of vegetable rich in vitamin C
- two other servings of vegetables including potato

The vegetables listed below may be served whole, whilst others can be chopped, sliced or grated; cold, raw, or hot by steaming, boiling, dry baking, dry roasting and seasoned with the following herbs and spices.

Artichokes: bayleaf, coriander, paprika and parsley
Asparagus: dill, marjoram, nutmeg and rosemary
Avocado: coriander, garlic, mustard and paprika
Beans (green): basil, dill, garlic and mustard
Beetroot (beets): chives, cloves, coriander, dill, ginger and thyme
Broccoli: garlic, marjoram and nutmeg
Brussels sprouts: carraway seeds, marjoram, nutmeg, oregano, parsley and rosemary
Cabbage: bayleaf, chives, curry, marjoram, nutmeg and parsley
Carrots: chives, curry, parsley, marjoram and nutmeg
Cauliflower: basil, curry, dill, ginger, rosemary, mint and coriander
Cucumber: basil, chives, dill, mustard and rosemary
Eggplant: basil, curry, garlic, parsley and rosemary
Leeks: bayleaf, dill, mustard, paprika and thyme
Lettuce: basil, chives, dill, garlic, rosemary, tarragon and thyme
Mushrooms: coriander, chives, curry, nutmeg, parsley, rosemary and thyme
Onions: basil, coriander, garlic, marjoram and paprika
Peas: basil, marjoram, mint, nutmeg, parsley and sage
Potatoes: chives, garlic, marjoram and paprika

Silverbeet (swiss chard): basil, bayleaf, coriander, garlic, marjoram, nutmeg, rosemary and sage
Tomatoes: basil, dill, chives, fennel, garlic, oregano, paprika, parsley, tarragon and thyme
Zucchini (courgettes): basil, garlic, oregano and parsley

Did you know?
Soaking prepared fresh vegetables leaches out the water-soluble vitamins and minerals into the liquid? If you soak vegetables at any time, always use the liquid as a stock for soup; do not throw it down the sink.

Vegetables and main meals, without meat

The days of overcooked, soggy vegetables are gone. Today the variety, texture and choices are almost endless. Modern cooking methods e.g., steaming and microwaving, produce vegetables that retain their colour, vitamins and minerals. New technology now means that many vegetable varieties can be offered through supermarkets and greengrocers virtually all year round.

Serve fresh vegetables that are minimally cooked. Overcooked vegetables will have lost their nutrients. Liberal use of herbs, spices and sauces, see pages 107 and 71 ff., will enhance the flavour and add dash to vegetable casseroles. Carefully wash and dry *all* vegetables before using. The different combinations of vegetables for stews and casseroles are unlimited in their methods of cooking:

Steaming	Stir 'frying'	Roasting
Dry baking	Boiling	Microwaving

Baked stuffed potatoes

6 large old potatoes, scrubbed and washed, but leave skin on

Preheat oven to 200°C. Dry bake potatoes on a rack in a hot oven until cooked.

filling
1 cup ricotta cheese, low fat
1 cup fresh corn kernels
½ fresh chives, chopped
mashed potato flesh
½ teaspoon dill
½ teaspoon nutmeg
freshly ground pepper
dash herb salt

Cut round hole in top of potato, scoop out flesh, and mash with all other ingredients. Carefully spoon mixture back into potato shells. Bake for a further 10 minutes in a hot oven. Remove, sprinkle with paprika and serve immediately. Potatoes can also be served cold.

Serves 4.

Baked sweet potatoes

2 orange sweet potatoes, medium size

Preheat oven to 250°C. Wash potatoes well and dry bake whole on a rack in a hot oven for approximately 35–40 minutes.

When ready to serve, slice and sprinkle with freshly ground pepper and nutmeg and arrange on serving platter.

Serves 4.

Barbecued vegetables in foil

Most vegetables are suitable, but here are a few suggestions.

enough potatoes for 4 serves
sprinkle of nutmeg
freshly ground pepper
quantity of foil

Wash and dry the potatoes, leave the skins on. With a sharp knife, slice the potatoes thinly and arrange side by side in the foil. Top with the herbs. Cover and place on the barbecue and cook until tender.

variations
Sweet potato, carrots (especially the Dutch variety, whole), or pumpkin (very thinly sliced).

Sweet potatoes, particularly the orange variety, are very versatile. Use them boiled, steamed, mashed or make them into puddings, desserts or cakes.

Broccoli, mushroom and onion toss

500 g broccoli, washed and broken into flowerettes
2 rashers chopped bacon — optional (rind and fat removed)
1 onion, peeled and finely chopped
125 g button mushrooms, sliced
½ cup white wine *or*
¼ cup grapefruit *or* lemon juice
½ teaspoon chilli sauce (optional)
freshly ground pepper

Steam, microwave, or blanch broccoli in boiling water for 3–5 minutes until cooked. Heat pan, add chopped bacon and onion and sauté until cooked. Add mushrooms, cook 1 minute, tossing gently. Add white wine or juice with chilli sauce, stir through. Add broccoli, cook 2 minutes, add a little pepper and serve.

Serves 4.

Cabbage rolls

Squeeze the cabbage rolls in a tea towel to give firmer shape and better looking rolls.

6 large cabbage leaves, firm and fresh
1½ cups fresh tomato sauce, recipe page 75
1 cup brown rice, cooked
½ cup fresh parsley, chopped
1 large onion, finely chopped
½ cup toasted pinenuts
dash herb salt
freshly ground pepper

Cook rice in 2 cups water, bring to boil and simmer until all water is absorbed and rice is cooked. (This can be done the day before, or left-over rice is suitable.)

Preheat the oven to 230°C. Blanch cabbage leaves in boiling water, one at a time, for 1 minute and drain on a tea towel; lay flat. Lightly sauté onion, add to rice with parsley, pinenuts, herb salt and pepper; mix through. Place a large spoonful of rice into each cabbage leaf and carefully roll up. Place in casserole dish, top with tomato sauce and bake in the oven for 20 minutes.

Serves 4–6.

Cauliflower sauté (Greek style)

The cooking time for this recipe will vary depending on how you like your vegetables; well cooked, medium cooked, or just lightly cooked.

½ cauliflower, broken into small flowerettes
2 medium size brown onions, sliced
2 cloves garlic, finely chopped
2 tablespoons tomato paste
½ teaspoon oregano
freshly ground pepper
½ cup white wine *or* ½ cup vegetable stock

Brush a heavy based pan or a wok with a little olive oil. Lightly sauté garlic and onions until brown and soft. Add cauliflower and stir in tomato paste and oregano. Add white wine or stock, stir and cover, simmer for 5 minutes. Add a little freshly ground pepper and serve as an accompaniment to meat or chicken. If preferred, you can cook all the ingredients in a teflon pan, but omit the olive oil. Cover and simmer for 5–7 minutes.

Serves 4.

Curried potatoes, carrots and peas

1 kg new potatoes, small
2 medium carrots, peeled and diced into cubes
2 cups fresh shelled peas *or* frozen peas
1 teaspoon curry powder
½ teaspoon cumin
½ teaspoon turmeric
1 teaspoon fennel seeds
freshly ground pepper
¼ cup vegetable stock, recipe page 25

Cut potatoes in half and steam or boil until not quite cooked. Heat wok or large pan and brush base with light olive oil. Add fennel seeds, cook 1 minute; add curry powder, cumin and turmeric. Then add potatoes and carrots; toss 1 minute, add stock and cook 5 minutes. Add the peas, cook a further 2 minutes and serve immediately.

Serves 4.

Curried mixed vegetables with snow peas and cashews

1 cup broccoli flowerettes
1 cup cauliflower flowerettes
1 large carrot *or* 2 small carrots, peeled, sliced diagonally
1 medium zucchini, sliced (ends removed)
1 large brown onion, chopped
1 celery stalk, washed, sliced diagonally
2 cloves garlic, minced *or* finely chopped
⅛ cabbage, finely shredded *or* 1½–2 cups
200 g snow peas (topped and tailed)
½ cup cashews, raw
½ teaspoon cumin
½ teaspoon ground coriander
½ teaspoon turmeric
1 heaped teaspoon curry powder
1 cup water
2 tablespoons light olive oil

Heat oil in wok, add garlic and onion and sauté until golden and soft. Add spices and curry powder, cook a further 2 minutes. Add all vegetables except snow peas and cabbage. Cook 2 minutes, tossing the vegetables regularly. Add water and cook another 5 minutes. Finally, add snow peas, cabbage and nuts; toss again, cook 3–5 minutes. Serve immediately from wok in centre of table accompanied with steamed brown rice.

Serves 4–6.

Eggplant preparation

Wash eggplant, and depending on how you intend to use it, cut in half and sprinkle liberally with salt. Leave standing for approximately 30–40 minutes. Wash salt off with water or wipe with cloth and gently squeeze eggplant to remove bitter juices.

Eggplant and mushroom stir 'fry'

2 medium eggplant, peeled and diced into cubes
300 g mushrooms, washed and sliced
1 small brown onion, peeled and chopped
2 cloves garlic, crushed *or* finely chopped
½ green pepper, chopped
½ red pepper, chopped
1 tablespoon tamari *or* soy sauce, low salt
1 tablespoon fresh parsley, chopped
½ teaspoon oregano
sprig fresh thyme
freshly ground pepper

Prepare eggplant, method as above, but for this recipe, peel first, salt well and leave to stand. Wash salt off after 30 minutes and squeeze out any further juices.

Heat about 1 tablespoon olive oil in a wok and sauté onion and garlic 3–5 minutes. Add eggplant, green and red pepper and sliced mushrooms, cook for a further 5 minutes stirring the wok occasionally. Add tamari, oregano, thyme, parsley and pepper, toss through. Cook for a further 5 minutes on high heat, making sure ingredients do not stick or burn. Serve immediately with rice and green salad.

Serves 4–6.

‘Battered’ eggplant

2 large eggplant, sliced, (prepared as shown)

batter
1 cup evaporated skim milk
1 egg white, beaten
½ teaspoon dried tarragon *or* 1 teaspoon fresh tarragon, chopped
½ teaspoon dried thyme *or* 1 teaspoon fresh thyme, chopped

After eggplant has been salted, washed and dried, slice, with the skin on ready to dip in batter. Mix all ingredients for batter. Dip eggplant in batter and cook in hot teflon coated pan or heavy based pan, brushed with light olive oil. Remember to turn eggplant over to other side when batter is cooked on one side.

Serves 4–6.

Leeks, carrots and celery

1 leek, cleaned thoroughly, and sliced
2 celery stalks, sliced
1 medium carrot, peeled, cut in half lengthways and sliced
2 tablespoons vegetable stock
½ teaspoon thyme
freshly ground pepper

Brush a saucepan with a little light olive oil and gently sauté leeks until tender. Add carrot, celery, thyme and pepper with the stock. Cover and simmer 5 minutes.

If preferred, you can omit olive oil. Gently cook leeks in stock until tender; add carrots, celery, thyme and pepper. Cook covered 5 minutes. (You may need to add a little more stock.)

Serves 4.

Plain omelette

1 egg
2 egg whites
1 tablespoon fresh parsley, chopped, *or*
1 tablespoon chives, chopped
freshly ground pepper
dash herb salt

Beat eggs with a fork in a small bowl. Add parsley, chives, ground pepper and herb salt. Heat a nonstick small pan until hot. Add egg mix, stir with fork, easing sides of omelette towards the centre with a nonstick spatula.

variations

Mushroom and chive omelette

Recipe as plain omelette. Add ¼ cup buttom mushrooms, sliced.

Vegetable omelette

Recipe as plain omelette but *add*
¼ cup carrot, grated
1 tablespoon cheese, low fat *or* parmesan, freshly grated

Chicken and chive omelette

Recipe as plain omelette. Add 1 tablespoon cooked chicken (no skin).

Tomato omelette

Recipe as plain omelette. Add 1 tomato, peeled and sliced.

Serves 1.

Pumpkin timbales

This recipe makes a superb entrée, particularly when served with a colourful ricotta sauce, low fat, recipe page 78

1 cup cooked pumpkin, mashed
½ small onion, chopped
½ cup cheese, low fat, grated, *or* parmesan, freshly grated
1 tablespoon nonfat yoghurt
2 egg whites
pinch nutmeg
freshly ground pepper

Preheat oven to 190°C. Heat a small pan lightly brushed with olive oil, or nonstick pan, and cook the onions until soft. Place all the ingredients with the onion into a blender and mix well. Spoon into 3 very small or 2 slightly larger baking dishes (lightly brushed with olive oil). Place the timbales into a tray about ¼ filled with warm water and bake in the oven about 15 minutes or until set. Remove the cooked timbale by running a heated knife around the edge of the dish and carefully turning out on to a plate. Timbales may be served either hot or cold topped with a ricotta sauce, low in fat.

variations

Cauliflower timbales

Recipe as above. Omit the pumpkin and add 1 cup of steamed cauliflowerettes and a pinch of curry powder.

Spinach or broccoli timbales

Recipe as above. Omit the pumpkin and add 1 cup of cooked spinach, *or* 1 cup steamed broccoli flowerettes.

Serves 2.

Sesame broccoli

500 g broccoli flowerettes, large

sauce
1 tablespoon tahini
1 tablespoon tamari *or* soy sauce, low salt
1 teaspoon honey
juice 1 lemon
1 tablespoon toasted sesame seeds

Steam or microwave broccoli until just tender. Arrange on serving platter. Blend all ingredients for sauce, pour over broccoli, then sprinkle with toasted sesame seeds.

Serves 4.

Steamed vegetables with yoghurt and herb dressing

Any steamed vegetables of your choice e.g., broccoli, cauliflower, beans, squash, zucchini, pumpkin etc.

dressing
1 cup nonfat yoghurt
1 tablespoon chives, chopped
1 dessertspoon fresh mint, chopped
juice ½ fresh lemon *or* lime
freshly ground pepper

Blend all ingredients. Serve separately in a jug and pour over the steamed vegetables.

Serves 4.

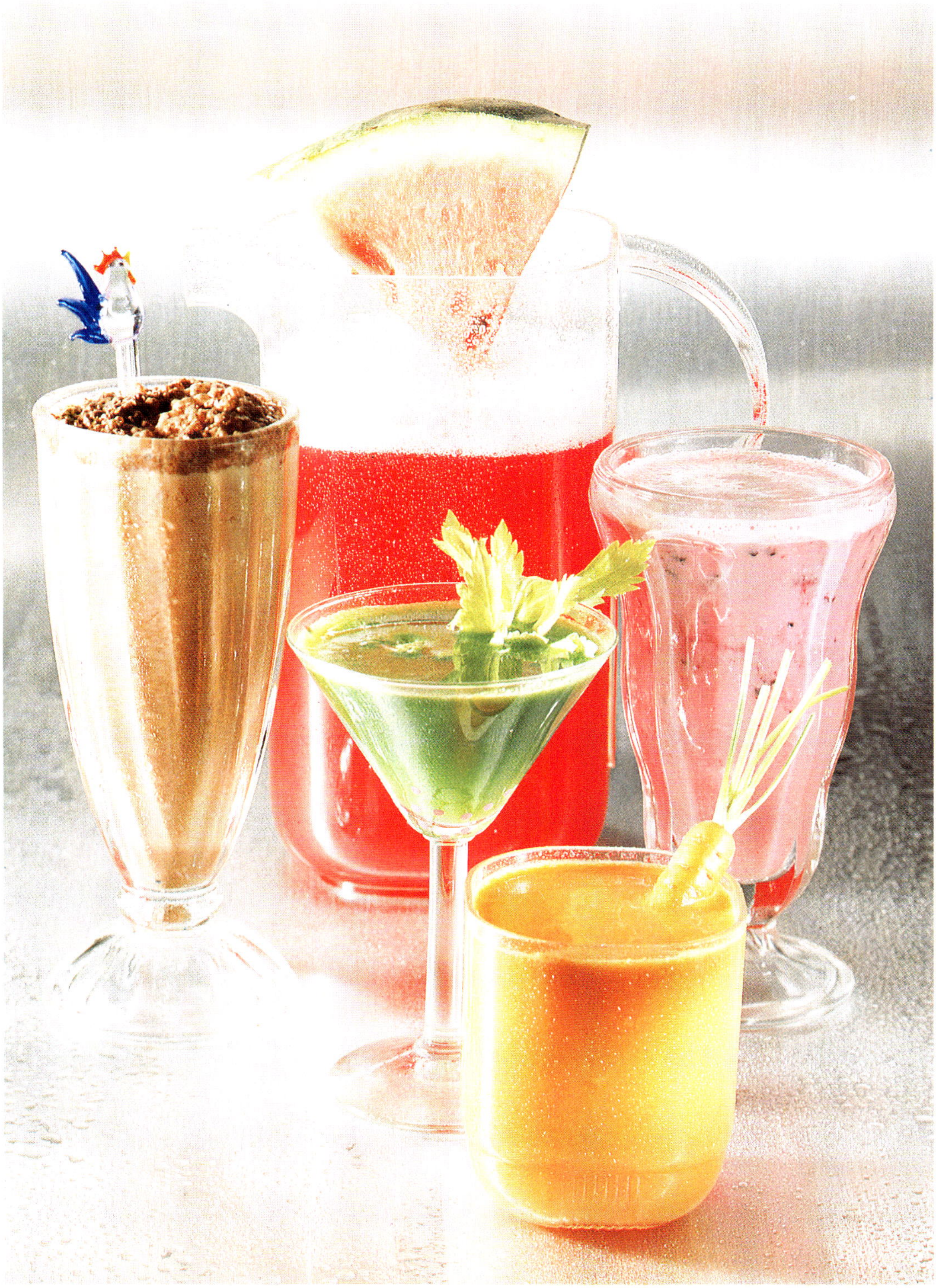

Watermelon delight (*page 143*), Banana health shake (*page 140*)
Cucumber, celery and parsley (*page 125*), Carrot and apple juice (*page 126*)
Raspberry delight with blackberries (*page 142*)

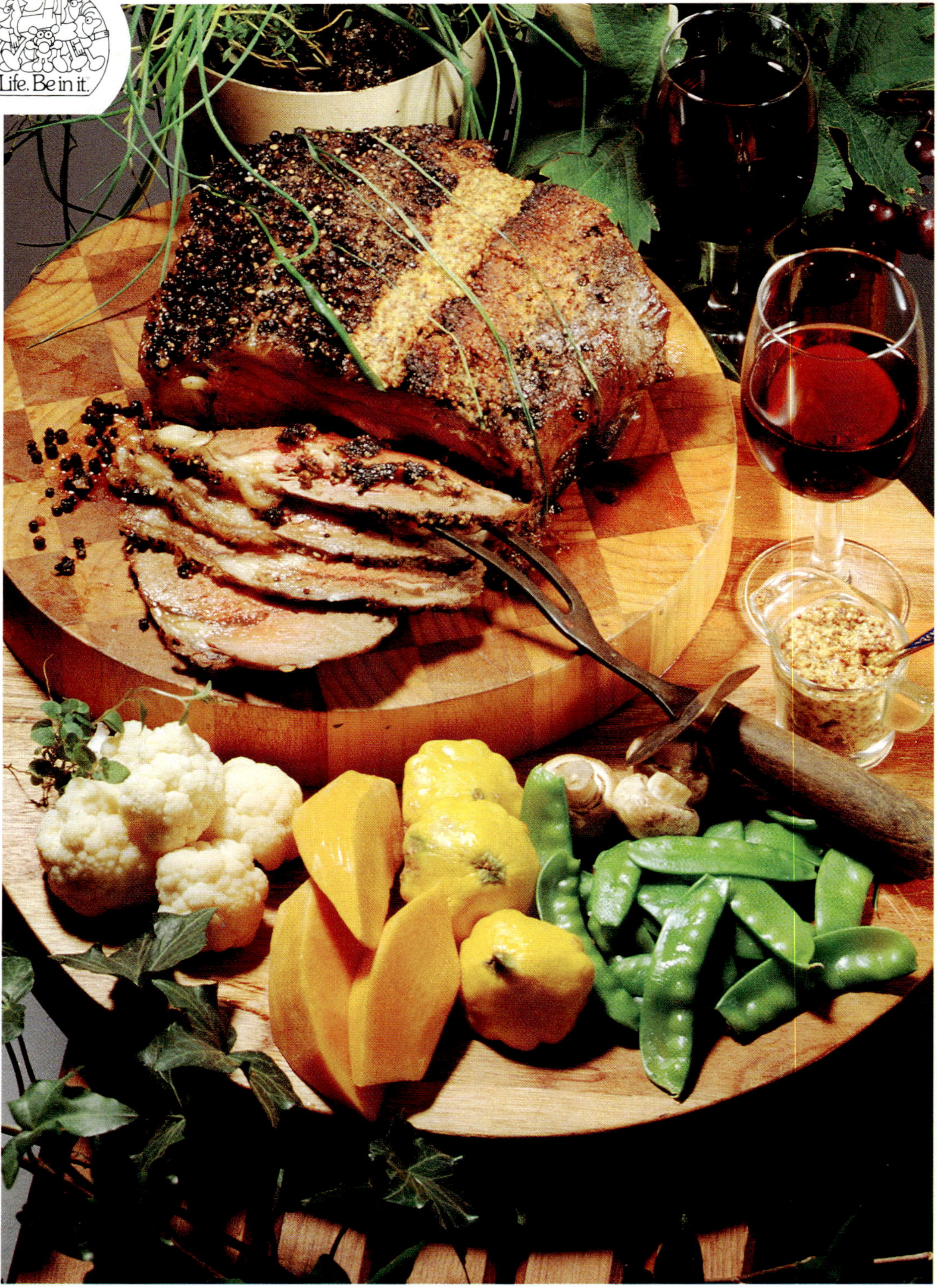

Roast boned sirloin beef (*page 42*)
Mixed steamed vegetables (*page 118*)
Berry juice surprise (*page 140*)

Stir 'fried' bananas

5 bananas, peeled and sliced
1 onion, finely chopped
4 tomatoes, peeled and chopped
3 tablespoons dry white wine
1 tablespoon soy sauce, low salt (optional)
generous pinch cayenne pepper

Gently sauté the onion in a nonstick pan (lid on), until tender. Add the remaining ingredients, carefully tossing the bananas and tomatoes for about 10 minutes.

Serves 4.

Vegetable 'burgers'

2 large potatoes, peeled and grated
1 large carrot, peeled and grated
3 spring onions, finely chopped
½ cup parsley, freshly chopped
½ cup grated cheese, low fat
2 eggs
2 egg whites
½ teaspoon curry powder
freshly ground pepper

Whisk eggs and whites together. Add all other ingredients and mix. Heat a nonstick frypan or a pan lightly brushed with light olive oil until hot. Place spoonfuls of mixture into pan and cook until golden on one side; turn and cook other side.

Makes about 6–8.

Vegetarian cannelloni

If time is a problem, you can buy cannelloni tubes, rather than making the crêpes. However, the result is not quite as good and the cooking time takes 15 minutes longer.

8–10 wholemeal crêpes, recipe page 95

filling
500 g fresh ricotta cheese, low fat
1 cup cooked spinach, chopped
½ cup fresh chives, chopped
½ cup fresh parsley, chopped
½ cup toasted pinenuts
½ teaspoon dill
½ teaspoon nutmeg
1 teaspoon basil
freshly ground pepper

topping
1½ cups fresh tomato sauce, recipe page 75
1½ cups skim milk white sauce, recipe page 80
grated cheese, low fat

Mix all the filling ingredients and place a large spoonful of the mixture on to the centre of each crêpe. Carefully roll up. Treat each crêpe in the same manner and place in a single layer on an oblong nonstick dish, or a dish lightly brushed with olive oil. Spoon over the tomato sauce and the skim milk white sauce alternately, so they will mix. Sprinkle with a little of the grated cheese and bake in a moderately hot oven for about 30 minutes.

Serves 4–5.

Vegetarian lasagne

Here is a delicious recipe for lasagne where we substitute azuki beans for meat.

500 g lasagne pasta
azuki bolognaise sauce, recipe page 72
skim milk white sauce, recipe page 80
¼ cup grated cheese, low fat
¼ cup parmesan, freshly grated
fresh tomato sauce, recipe page 75

Prepare the azuki bolognaise and white sauce according to recipe. Boil water in a large pot, add 1 teaspoon olive oil. Cook pasta sheets (3–4 at a time), until just cooked. *Do not overcook*. Remove carefully, drain and run under cold water. Spread out on a dry tea towel.

Preheat oven to 180°C. Brush a not too wide, but deep baking dish with a little olive oil. Place a layer of pasta in bottom of the dish. Cover with a thin layer of white sauce; spread a layer of azuki bolognaise sauce, then another layer of pasta. Continue until sauce and pasta have all been used. Sprinkle top with half-and-half cheeses and bake in the oven 30–40 minutes.

Serves 4.

When selecting cheese — look for the reduced salt-hard and low in fat varieties. They are great as toppings in sauces or can be served grated in sandwiches or on salads.

Vegetable soufflé

Good results are achieved when cooking a soufflé by placing it in a baking dish half filled with hot water. This spreads the heat evenly and prevents drying out.

1½ cups broccoli flowerettes
1½ cups cauliflower flowerettes
2 large carrots, peeled and chopped
1 parsnip, peeled and chopped
1 dessertspoon curry powder
1 teaspoon cumin
¼ teaspoon nutmeg
little margarine
freshly ground pepper
4 egg whites

Preheat oven to 220°C. Steam broccoli, cauliflower, carrots and parsnip until tender. Purée in blender. Sauté curry powder, cumin, nutmeg and pepper in pan with a little margarine for approximately 2 minutes to bring out the flavour. Add to puréed vegetables and stir through. Lightly grease 6 small or 1 large soufflé dish. Beat egg whites until stiff and carefully fold through the cooled puréed vegetables. Pour into soufflé dishes and bake approximately 20 minutes until golden and fluffy. Serve with tahini and yoghurt sauce, recipe page 82.

Serves 4–6.

Dark green leafy vegetables are a source of calcium, fibre and vitamins A and C. It is better to buy them fresh or grow your own and eat as soon as possible, minimally cooked.

Wholemeal vegetable pie

To prevent the white sauce from thinning whilst cooking, it is important to use a very thick white sauce. This will stop the sauce from spilling out of the pie.

1 quantity wholemeal pastry, recipe page 69 *or* 2–3 sheets wholemeal shortcrust pastry (ready rolled)
2 medium potatoes, peeled and quartered
250 g pumpkin, peeled and cut into chunks
½ cup broccoli pieces
½ cup cauliflower pieces
1 small zucchini sliced
1 carrot, peeled and sliced
freshly chopped basil
dash herb salt
freshly ground pepper
while sauce (thick), recipe page 83

Steam all vegetables until tender. (Zucchini, broccoli and cauliflower will not take as long as other vegetables.)

Preheat oven to 190°C. Use a 20 cm × 8 cm nonstick tin or lightly grease with olive oil. Line whole of the tin (base and sides), with wholemeal pastry. Arrange vegetables in tin and sprinkle with basil, herb salt and freshly ground pepper. Pour over thick white sauce. Cover top with remaining pastry, brush with egg white and make a few holes for the steam to escape. Bake in the oven for approximately 35–40 minutes until pastry is a golden colour. If preferred, instead of a pastry cover, grated cheese can be sprinkled over entire top of pie together with poppy seeds and a little paprika, and baked as above.

Serves 4–6.

Zucchini and potato frittata

1 medium–large potato, peeled and thinly sliced
2 small zucchini, thinly sliced
4 egg whites
2 tablespoons milk, low fat
1 teaspoon parmesan cheese, freshly grated
1 tablespoon fresh chives, chopped
dash herb salt
freshly ground pepper

Brush a small pan with light olive oil or a nonstick pan and heat to hot. Add sliced potato, cook 2 minutes. Add zucchini, toss gently, then cook further for 1 minute. Beat egg whites and milk lightly with a fork, add parmesan cheese, chives, salt and pepper and pour over vegetables in pan. Reduce heat and cook gently until mixture sets. Loosen carefully, turn on to serving plate, cut into wedges, and serve with tossed green salad.

variation

Sweet corn and capsicum frittata

Recipe as above. Omit the zucchini and use:
2 corn cobs (fresh)
1 red capsicum
1 green capsicum

Remove corn by slicing from cob. Cut capsicums in half, seed, and cut into fine thin strips. Cook as above.

Serves 2.

Vegetable juices

Vegetable drinks are made by extracting the natural juices from a variety of vegetables which provide vitamins and minerals and quench the thirst. They also give an energy boost. There are many combinations from which you can choose so experiment with your own juice extractor. Choose vegetables that are fresh and, where possible, home grown are the best. Old or wilted vegetables have no vitamins. Most juices are suitable; however, exercise a little caution when drinking carrot juice — too much may cause vitamin A toxicity. Most vegetable juices are usually too strong to drink undiluted so add water or combine with other juices for a satisfactory result. They may be consumed any time of the day and are usually served cold or over ice. Remember, wash and dry the vegetables carefully, before using.

Cucumber, celery and parsley

3 celery stalks, washed and cut into pieces
½ cucumber peeled and cut into pieces
½ bunch parsley, well washed

Combine the vegetables, put through the juice extractor and pour into glasses. If desired, pour over crushed ice.

variation

Cucumber, celery and apple

Recipe as above. Omit the parsley and add 2 apples, peeled and chopped.

Serves 3–4.

Carrot and apple juice

1 kg carrots, washed and cut into pieces
3–4 apples, peeled and quartered

Process the carrot and apple through the juice extractor and pour into glasses. If desired, pour over crushed ice. Drink immediately for optimum nutritional value.

variation

Carrot, celery and apple juice

Recipe as above.
Add 1 cup celery, chopped

Serves 4–6.

Salads

Salads, using fresh, raw, well washed vegetables preferably straight from the garden, contain the highest source of vitamins, minerals and fibre. Select and combine vegetables with grains, wholemeal pasta and fruits according to taste and preference. The whole family can participate when making up salads. Let your imagination run wild! There are some exquisite combinations, especially when chosen for colour and appearance which will also satisfy the appetite. Remember: wash and dry all vegetables carefully before using.

Tips and hints

- ice cold water will revive carrots, lettuce, cauliflower and celery
- refrigerate and use cold ingredients, except if the salad is hot
- do not soak vegetables as the water-soluble vitamins will leak into the liquid

Avocado, grapefruit and melon salad

1 mignonnette lettuce, washed and well drained
1 large avocado, ripe
1 grapefruit, skinned and cut into sections — keep any juice to rub on avocado
½ ripe cantaloup *or* honey dew melon
Quantity of chive dressing, recipe page 74

Arrange lettuce pieces in a bowl. Cut avocado in half. Peel off skin and slice into long thin slices. Peel cantaloup and slice in the same manner and place in alternate layers in the bowl. Sprinkle grapefruit segments on salad, mix dressing and pour over prior to serving.

Serves 4.

Avocado salad with lime and yoghurt dressing

3 or 4 ripe avocados
½ red spanish onion, finely sliced
½ bunch radishes, finely sliced
12 black olives
1 tablespoon fresh chives, chopped
½ cup lime and yoghurt dressing, recipe page 77

Peel and slice avocados and lime and place on a serving platter. Sprinkle the onion rings, radishes and olives on top. Pour over the dressing. Sprinkle with chopped chives.

Serves 4–6.

Broccoli, snow pea and pinenut salad

3 cups broccoli flowerettes, washed
350 g snow peas, (ends removed)
2 tablespoons pinenuts

Blanch broccoli and snow peas in boiling water for 1 minute. Remove, place under cold water to refresh, then drain and set aside. Refrigerate until ready to serve.

Combine a dressing of 1 tablespoon light olive oil, 1 clove garlic finely chopped, 1 tablespoon cider vinegar or juice of ½ lemon, and ½ teaspoon Dijon mustard. When ready to serve, place vegetables in bowl, toast pinenuts in heavy based pan on high heat, add to salad and pour dressing over. Serve immediately.

Serves 4.

Tofu, is a product of the soya bean. It is relatively high in protein and may be added to salads or mixed with fruit.

Carrot salad with dressing

3 large carrots, grated
1 cup raisins *or* sultanas
½ cup walnuts, chopped
12 cherry tomatoes

dressing
1½ tablespoons light olive oil
juice of 1 large lemon
½ teaspoon coriander
rind of 1 lemon, finely grated
freshly ground pepper

Place the carrots, raisins and tomatoes in a serving bowl. Mix the dressing ingredients. Pour over the salad and toss. Top with the walnuts and chill.

Serves 4.

Cauliflower salad with soy and yoghurt dressing

½ small cauliflower divided into flowerettes and blanched in boiling water for 4 minutes. Run under cold water and drain
125 g snow peas, blanched 1 minute in boiling water. Run under cold water and drain
½ bunch radishes, trimmed and sliced *or* quartered
1 red Spanish onion, thinly sliced
quantity of soy and yoghurt dressing, recipe page 82

Combine all vegetables and pour over the dressing.

Serves 4.

Life. Be in it.

Coleslaw

¼ crisp fresh cabbage (half white cabbage, half red cabbage)
½ green pepper, cut in half again and thinly sliced
1 carrot, peeled and grated
3 spring onions, finely chopped

Wash red and white cabbage, dry and drain on a tea towel. Shred thinly and place in a bowl. Add grated carrot, chopped spring onions and sliced green pepper.

dressing
In a small jar put: 1 tablespoon soy mayonnaise
1 tablespoon cider vinegar
freshly ground pepper

Mix, pour over salad and toss.

Serves 4–6.

Herbed bean and sesame salad

500 g fresh beans (topped and tailed by hand)
sesame seeds, toasted
quantity of herbed French dressing, recipe page 76

Steam beans until just tender. *Do not overcook.* Refresh under running water, pat dry. Pour the dressing over the beans and top with the sesame seeds.

Serves 4.

Orange and watercress salad

3 sweet oranges, in season
1 small red onion, thinly sliced
1 bunch of fresh, young, watercress

dressing
1 tablespoon light olive oil
juice of ½ lemon
dash of herb salt

Peel and cut the oranges into slices. Remove the pith. Trim the watercress, if necessary, and arrange on to a serving platter. Place the orange slices on top of the watercress. Mix the dressing ingredients and pour over the salad.

Serves 4.

Spinach salad

½ bunch spinach
1 red onion, thinly sliced
1 cup mushrooms, sliced
1 cup cucumber, peeled and thinly sliced
½ cup walnuts, chopped
toasted sesame seeds
quantity of tamari and honey dressing, recipe page 82

Wash spinach well (at least 4 or 5 times). Break leaves into pieces in a salad bowl. Add the onion rings, sliced fresh mushrooms, cucumber and walnuts. Mix dressing ingredients and pour over salad when ready to serve. Sprinkle with toasted sesame seeds.

Serves 4.

Tofu and tamari salad

8–10 cubes fresh tofu (soy bean curd)
¼ cup tamari *or* soy sauce, low salt

garnish
¼ cup chives, chopped
1 spring onion, chopped
finely grated ginger

Arrange the cubes of tofu on a serving platter. Pour the tamari over the tofu. Top with the onions and ginger. Serve with extra tamari in a separate bowl beside the platter.

Serves 4.

Potato salad

5 medium red potatoes, skin on
5 spring onions
1 tablespoon fresh chives, chopped
handful fresh parsley, chopped
quantity of tarragon and yoghurt dressing, recipe page 83

Scrub potatoes well, steam until tender then cut into chunks (skin on). Place into a large bowl. Top with the chives and parsley and pour over the dressing.

Serves 4–6.

Tossed mixed green salad

½ butter lettuce
½ mignonnette lettuce } well washed, drained and dried in colander *or* salad spinner
3 spring onions, washed and finely chopped
2 celery stalks, washed and finely chopped
1 medium green pepper, seeded and finely chopped
⅓ Italian cucumber, peeled and diced
½ cup parsley, finely chopped and well washed
½ avocado (skin removed), thinly sliced and cut into pieces

Break lettuce into small pieces with your hands, into a large bowl. Add spring onions, celery, green pepper, cucumber, parsley and avocado.

This salad is delicious with either soy and yoghurt dressing, recipe page 82, *or* herbed French dressing, recipe page 76. Pour over just prior to serving and toss.

Serves 4.

Tossed mixed salad

lettuce leaf-lined salad bowl
¼ lettuce, washed, drained, torn into bite-size pieces
1 carrot cut into julienne strips
4 button mushrooms, sliced
2 radishes, thinly sliced
¼ cup nonfat yoghurt

Prepare all the ingredients, toss very gently and place into the lined bowl. Chill and top with the yoghurt. Serve as an accompaniment to a barbecue or your favourite meat.

Serves 4.

Fruit

The joys of summer bring an abundance of fresh fruit. What better way to enjoy fruit than eaten freshly picked from the tree or vine?

Fruit is an excellent source of vitamin C, providing valuable roughage and natural sugars in the diet. Vitamin A is also present in some fruits.

Vitamin C sources.
Oranges, lemons, strawberries, grapefruit, kiwi fruit, raspberries, gooseberries and loganberries.

Vitamin A sources (small amounts only).
Apricots, peaches and tomatoes.

Dried fruits in particular, add flavour to both sweet and savoury recipes, providing fibre and energy. Satisfy the family or guests by serving a superb fruit salad made from selected choice fruit combinations at the conclusion of a meal. Everyone will enjoy it.

For a healthy diet, eat at least once every day:

- one serving of vitamin C fruit
- two other servings of fruit

Sultanas and raisins, although almost the same, come from different varieties of grapes. They are a good source of fibre and natural sugar (fructose). Use them to sweeten desserts or add that extra flavour to a salad.

Fruit salads and desserts

Fruit salads and desserts are a delightful and refreshing way to conclude a good meal. Many of the seasonal fruits, except berries and some stone fruits, are now available almost all year round. Use natural fruit juices and concentrates, or dried fruits such as dates, sultanas and raisins. Serve hot or cold with your favourite nonfat yoghurt, ricotta cheese, low in fat or fruit sauces. They are all low in fat and may prevent the waistline from expanding. It is quite permissible to use fruits canned in their natural juices as a base for fruit salads and desserts. Remember; always wash carefully, dry, and remove the skin where necessary before using.

Baked apples with dates, banana and walnuts

4 large Granny Smith apples (in season)
1 small ripe banana, sliced and cut in half again
3 or 4 dates, chopped
½ cup walnuts, chopped
cinnamon
4 tablespoons fresh orange juice
extra orange juice

Wash and core apples (leave skin on). Put apples into small baking dish and fill with a mixture of banana, dates and walnuts. Sprinkle with cinnamon and pour orange juice over top of each apple. Bake in moderate oven 40–50 minutes. Half way through cooking, pour a little extra orange juice over apples and add an extra dash of cinnamon.

Serve warm with spoonful of nonfat yoghurt.

Serves 4.

Barbecued or baked whole bananas

6–8 ripe bananas, whole, skins left on

Barbecue

Wash and dry the skins of the bananas and place them on to the barbecue plate or grill. Turn bananas over as each side cooks or when they begin to blacken. To serve, carefully remove each banana from its skin and eat with your meat dishes or serve as a dessert.

Oven baked

Preheat the oven to 180°C.

Prepare as above and arrange the whole bananas on to a nonstick baking tray and place in the oven. Bake for about 20 minutes or until the bananas are cooked. Serve as above.

variation

Barbecued pineapple

Slices of fresh pineapple, quartered, skin left on

Place the pineapple pieces on to the barbecue plate and gently turn each slice over as it browns. Serve with either meat recipes or as a dessert.

Serves 4–6.

Blintzes

6–8 thin wholemeal crêpes, recipe page 95
a quantity of mango, plum and fig dessert, recipe page 138

Make up the filling and spread a portion on to each crêpe. Fold crêpes into quarters and pour over the remainder of the filling. Serve warm, topped with nonfat yoghurt.

variations
This recipe can be made with any of the following fillings you select to alter the flavour of the blintzes.

Orange ricotta sauce, recipe page 78

Ricotta and currant filling. Fold juice-soaked currants into ricotta cheese, low fat.

Marinate a selection of dried fruits of choice in fresh fruit juice.

Fresh orange juice with a dash of Cointreau and thickened with a small amount of arrowroot.

Raspberry sauce, recipe page 78

Serves 6–8.

Cantaloup and fresh fruit

1 cantaloup, cut into 8 slices
1 punnet fresh raspberries
2 kiwi fruit
bunch green *or* black grapes
1 banana (soaked in lemon juice)

Arrange 2 slices of cantaloup on each serving plate. Beside cantaloup, place a spoonful of remaining fruit (mixed). Decorate with a sprig of fresh mint and a spoonful of banana ricotta cream, recipe page 73, or orange ricotta sauce, recipe page 78, on side of serving plate.

Serves 4.

Fresh raspberry ice cream

1 punnet fresh raspberries *or* strawberries
375 g can evaported skim milk
2 tablespoons skim milk powder
½ cup apple juice concentrate
1 tablespoon gelatine

Dissolve gelatine in a little warm water and add to all other ingredients. Whip together in mixer or food processor. Freeze until ready to serve.

Serves 4.

Fresh strawberry and kiwi fruit crêpes

6–8 wholemeal crêpes, recipe page 95
1 punnet ripe strawberries, sliced
2 kiwi fruit, peeled and sliced
fresh orange juice

Place a mixture of strawberries and kiwi fruit in centre of each crêpe. Squeeze a little orange juice on the fruit and carefully fold in half, or roll up, whichever is preferred. Crêpes may be warmed in oven or served cold with natural yoghurt, low in fat and, if desired, fresh raspberry or strawberry sauce as well.

variation

Apple and sultana crêpes

6–8 wholemeal crêpes, recipe page 95
3 Granny Smith apples, peeled and sliced
¼ teaspoon cloves *or* 2 whole cloves
pinch nutmeg, freshly grated
1 tablespoon water

Place all the ingredients in a small saucepan and simmer gently until the apples are cooked. Set aside to cool. Place a spoonful of apples in centre of crêpe together with a dessertspoon of sultanas. Fold in half, or roll up. These may be served warmed in oven, or cold, with either nonfat yoghurt or orange ricotta sauce.

Serves 4–6.

Fruit kebabs

1 kiwi fruit, peeled and cut into chunks
6 black grapes, whole
1 banana, peeled and cut into 3 cm pieces
6 strawberries, hulled, whole
2 wooden skewers
pulp of two passionfruit

Thread the prepared fruit alternately on to each of the skewers. Top with the passionfruit. Refrigerate and serve as a breakfast or dessert.

Serves 2.

Fruit salads

Fruit salads may be made from a collection of fresh fruits of your choice or a mixture of fresh fruits and canned fruits in their natural juices. Here are some combinations I like. You may prefer to select your own.

Apples	Watermelon balls	Peaches
Pineapple	Cantaloup balls	Pears
Oranges	Oranges	Oranges
Kiwi fruit	Passionfruit	Passionfruit
Passionfruit		Strawberries

Serves 4–6.

Mango, plum and fig dessert

1 mango, peeled and chopped
6 plums, preferably dark red in colour, peeled and stoned
4 figs, fresh, chopped
½ cup apple juice concentrate
2 tablespoons arrowroot

Place the plums, figs and apple juice concentrate in a small saucepan and slowly simmer until soft. Thicken with the arrowroot and add the mango just before serving. This recipe can be used as a topping on pears, peaches and apples or with crêpes and blintzes.

Makes about 1–1½ cups.

Spiced fruiti grapefruit

2 grapefruit (yellow *or* pink), cut in half with spiked edges
1½ cups mixed fruit, chopped
1 tablespoon apple juice concentrate
½ teaspoon cinnamon

Place the grapefruit, spiked sides up, into 4 small bowls. Combine with the remaining ingredients. Divide the mixture into 4 and spoon equal amounts on to each grapefruit half. Serve as a breakfast or brunch.

Serves 4.

Peaches in raspberry sauce

4–6 whole peaches, lightly stewed *or* 12 peaches canned in their natural juice, drained
a quantity of raspberry sauce, recipe page 78

Place a peach or 2 halves into separate dessert bowls. Pour the sauce over the peaches and top with nonfat yoghurt.

Serves 4–6.

Stewed apples with orange ricotta sauce

4 Granny Smith apples, peeled and sliced
2 tablespoons water
¼ teaspoon ground cloves *or* 3–4 whole cloves
a little nutmeg, freshly grated
orange rind, freshly grated
1 quantity of orange ricotta sauce, recipe page 78

Place the apples, cloves, nutmeg and water in a saucepan and gently simmer until cooked. Set aside and cool. Prepare the orange ricotta sauce. Serve the apples into dessert dishes, remove the cloves and top with the sauce and grated orange rind.

Serves 4.

Fruit drinks

Homemade fruit drinks, served chilled, will satisfy the most jaded palate. They can be served as humble orange juices for breakfast or in their most exotic combinations to guests at dinner parties. It is not always necessary to serve alcohol. There is a high liquid content in fruit and their juice can be extracted very quickly. Use of a juice extractor will save precious time when you are in a hurry. Select fresh fruit. Always wash and dry the skin carefully before using. Remove the skin where necessary.

Banana health shake

2 cups skim milk
1 teaspoon wheatgerm
1–2 tablespoons carob powder
1 ripe banana
1 tablespoon nonfat yoghurt

Blend all ingredients. Serve in tall wide glasses and sprinkle with a little carob.

Serves 2–4.

Berry juice surprise

4 cups unsweetened apple juice
½ punnet blackberries
½ punnet strawberries
crushed ice (optional)

Put the blackberries and raspberries through a juice extractor. Strain if necessary. Combine the berry juice with the unsweetened apple juice. Chill and serve over crushed ice.

Makes about 5 cups.

Fruit salad punch

4 cups unsweetened apple juice
2 cups blood plums, stoned and juiced
2 cups fresh fruit salad, using fruits of choice
crushed ice (optional)

Combine the apple juice and juiced plums. Gently stir in the fruit salad. Serve over crushed ice.

Makes about 8 cups.

Orange apricot fiesta

4 cups orange juice, freshly squeezed
2 cups apricot nectar *or* juiced fresh apricots
1 kiwi fruit, peeled and finely chopped
crushed ice (optional)

garnish
kiwi fruit slices

Mix the juices, fruit and crushed ice. Garnish with the kiwi fruit slices and serve chilled.

Serves 4–6.

Vegetable and fruit purées make tasty sauce replacements to be served with meat recipes.

Life. Be in it.

Pineapple and orange julep

1 small ripe pineapple cut into pieces, (skin removed)
1½ cups orange juice, freshly squeezed

garnish
strawberries

Put pineapple through the juice extractor. Add to the orange juice, stir and serve topped with strawberries.

variation

Pineapple, orange and strawberry julep

Recipe as above. Add ½ punnet of fresh strawberries, washed and hulled, to the pineapple.

Serves 3–4.

Raspberry delight

½ punnet fresh raspberries
1½ cups orange juice, freshly squeezed
½ ripe banana
½ cup nonfat yoghurt
crushed ice (optional)

Blend all ingredients. Serve in tall glasses with a little crushed ice.

variation

Raspberry delight with blackberries

Recipe as above. Omit the orange juice and add 1½ cups skim milk powder and ½ cup blackberries just before the ingredients are blended. Only partly blend the blackberries.

Serves 3–4.

Tropical smoothie

½ small ripe pineapple (skin removed)
1 cup orange juice, freshly squeezed
1 ripe banana
½ cup nonfat yoghurt

Put pineapple through juice extractor and place in blender. Add orange juice, banana and yoghurt. Blend and pour immediately into tall glasses and serve.

Serves 4.

Watermelon delight

1 large piece of watermelon (skin removed)

garnish
sprigs of mint

Put the watermelon through the juice extractor. Pour into glasses and garnish with the mint.

variation

Spicy watermelon and apple delight

Recipe as above. Omit the sprigs of mint. Add 2 apples and ¼ teaspoon cinnamon.

Serves 3–4.

Index

Other books by the publishers

Suzanne Porter's keeping it low
Understanding cholesterol
Keeping it low with meat
The sweet alternative
Suzanne Porter's diets for low cholesterol day by day
Cooking naturally (Lowan wholefoods cookbook) Health stores
Old world cookbook (The old grain mill) Supermarkets